The CONFIDENT YOU

The CONFIDENT YOU

A Woman's Guide to Eternal Beauty

~

Barbara Barrington Jones
with Kris Mackay

Deseret Book Company
Salt Lake City, Utah

Library of Congress Cataloging-in-Publication Data

Jones, Barbara Barrington.
   The confident you : a guide to eternal beauty / Barbara Barrington
Jones with Kris Mackay.
     p.   cm.
   Includes index.
   ISBN 0-87579-604-4
   1. Beauty, Personal. I. Mackay, Kris. II. Title.
   RA778.J612   1992
   646.7'042—dc20   91-47723
                                             CIP

Printed in the United States of America   72082

10 9 8 7 6 5

Contents

vi   *Contents*

Preface

When a mutual friend brought us together and suggested that we collaborate on a book, we (Barbara and Kris) were intrigued. The friend said, "I've heard Barbara speak, and I've seen the hunger women have for what she has to offer. Let's make it available to all women."

The more we considered the possibility, the more enthusiastic we became. Perhaps by combining our specific skills, we could translate to the printed page the same excitement and motivation that Barbara generates in person.

We didn't take the assignment lightly. We began to travel together while Barbara spoke and Kris absorbed and analyzed the message and put it on paper. We interviewed numerous women as to their needs.

Last, but certainly not least, we knelt in prayer before every work session, beseeching the Lord for clarity of thought and expression and praying that somewhere within these pages you, the reader, would find fulfillment and peace.

Acknowledgments

My love and gratitude go to Ron Hills and Glen McClure, who work with the Church Educational System Youth and Family Programs. Proceeds from this book will go into a scholarship fund for summer youth camps at Brigham Young University.

I want to thank my wonderful husband, Hal Jones, whom I adore with all my heart. I thank him for his infinite wisdom, his love, his unending support, and his priceless time in helping me with this endeavor.

I also thank my sweet assistant, Lorie O'Toole, for her many hours of work and caring, and my dear friend Helen Wells for her beautiful contribution in chapter 5. And to the lovely ladies who allowed me to use their stories and photographs, I extend a debt of gratitude.

Kris and I thank our good friend and editor, Eleanor Knowles; without her, this book would never have been written. We are also grateful to Richard Erickson, designer of the book, and Patti Taylor, typographer.

We wish to thank the following persons for their help in their fields of expertise:

Russ Fischella of San Francisco, the country's leading glamour photographer.

Clark Smith of Los Angeles, professional photographer.

Barbara Palmer, one of the finest colorist/stylists in the San Francisco area.

Susan Davis, skin-care expert at La Costa Spa in San Diego.

Mica, a leading makeup artist at Coreen Cordoba Salon in San Francisco.

Ron Marquardt, Ph.D., director of nutrition and fitness for the Longevity Center in the San Francisco Bay area.

Larry Dietz, Ph.D., MFFC, who wrote his doctoral dissertation on self-esteem of working versus nonworking women.

Robert Read, M.D., for sharing information on P.M.S.

David Costanza, M.D., for his wisdom, caring, and compassion.

Foreword

By Kris Mackay

Before you read this book and begin your journey of self-improvement, let me acquaint you with the background of Barbara Barrington Jones and tell you why she is uniquely qualified to be your guide.

Perhaps you already know Barbara as a trainer of beauty queens, as the woman who helped to coach five Miss USAs in a row—the winners of the Miss USA beauty pageants from 1985 through 1989. Or you may be among the thousands who have heard her speak on the BYU Education Week or Especially for Youth circuits, since her conversion to The Church of Jesus Christ of Latter-day Saints in 1981.

The foundation for Barbara's direction in life was laid years ago by her mother, a model and fashion designer who could look at suits in *Vogue* magazine, cut patterns out of brown paper on the dining room table, and do a perfect job of tailoring them. By the time Barbara enrolled in kindergarten, she knew more about fashion and fabrics than she did about her ABCs. Her mother has always been Barbara's role model for the Confident Woman.

Barbara's consuming ambition as a child was to become a classical ballerina. She began practicing twirls and pliés when she was five, and by the age of nineteen her talents helped her to win a Miss America preliminary in the state of Texas. She studied ballet in New York and later performed with many prestigious companies. After she made her professional debut with the Atlanta Ballet Company, her career took her to Montreal and from there to teaching ballet at the University of Texas and the position of assistant artistic director of the University Ballet Company. After six months as guest teacher and choreographer of the Corpus Christi Civic Ballet Company, she started her own studio in El Paso.

Then Barbara branched out into acting. One day she auditioned for the part of Madame Dominique Beaurevears in the play *A Shot in the Dark*. The role called for her to be the richest woman in Paris, which Barbara definitely was not. But she wanted the role desperately. She went to a thrift shop and purchased a matching dress and cape for eight dollars and an old fur coat for not much more. She cut up the fur coat to trim the outfit, fashioned a muff from one sleeve, a stylish hat from the other, and covered the tops of her boots with parts of what was left.

She also prepared her mind to be the richest woman in Paris by determing to walk like Madame Beaurevears, talk like Madame Beaurevears, and be Madame Beaurevears. Because the role demanded it, she became (in her mind) rich, arrogant, flamboyant, and very, very confident. And she got the part.

Acting confirmed for Barbara that she could take control of how other people perceive her and, further, that the first step for any woman toward being attractive and confident is to think of herself as attractive and confident. Barbara learned to play other characters through her posture and movements. She could appear self-conscious or self-confident, rich or poor, sick or well, old or young. She believes that if we understand which movements portray aging, we can avoid some of those tell-tale postures in our later years.

She also modeled, not to make modeling a career but to make extra money. Modeling refined her poise in walking, sitting, standing, and knowing how to dress with flair.

With all that background, she went to work as a fashion designer for Guyrex Associates, a design firm that was affiliated with beauty pageants. Her jobs there were varied, ranging from helping to decorate floats to designing wigs and headpieces and helping to create gowns for theatrical productions and for state and national beauty queens. Working with Guyrex Associates taught her to be creative in all aspects of fashion.

After three years with the firm, she became director and administrator of the Barbizon School of Modeling in El Paso and, later, in Dallas. She prepared teachers who in turn trained students. This exposure taught her to bring out the best in each young woman, internally and externally, through building self-esteem while improving physical appearance.

The first year at Barbizon gave Barbara a brand new experience. For the first time in her life she sat behind a desk, still working from ten to twelve hours a day—but they were sedentary days. She developed headaches and stomachaches and over-ate in response to her sudden lack of exercise. That was when she began to develop her own exercise and eating programs.

After moving to San Francisco in 1976, Barbara accepted the position of fashion coordinator with Ghirardelli Square on the wharf, working with twenty-three fashion shops and presenting numerous fashion extravaganzas. There she learned to put together a wide variety of fashion designs for entertainment.

A ballet dancer, actress, fashion model, fashion designer, and coordinator must, of course, pay attention to her body in a way the average person normally does not. Barbara had to maintain a certain weight in order to have a job. But from all those years of training she acquired more valuable information, and she is committed to sharing what she learned. She believes that internal beauty is even more to be desired than the external kind, but they are both necessary for becoming The Confident You.

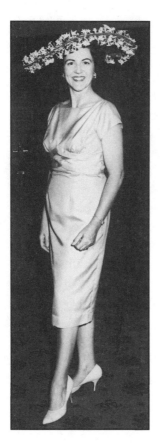

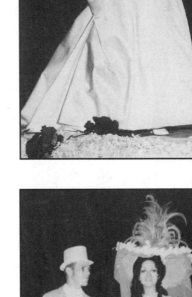

"*Above left:* It always pleased
me when people told me
that I resembled my mother.
Above right: Here is where
my affiliation and love for
pageants began. *Right:* My career as a dancer served me
well in the dramatic role of
Lady Boxington in *My Fair
Lady.*"

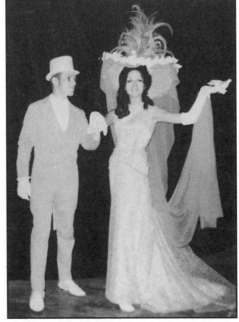

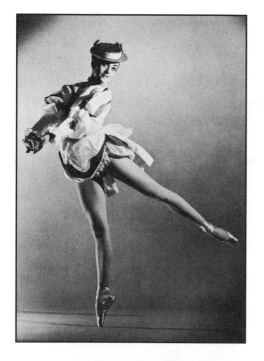

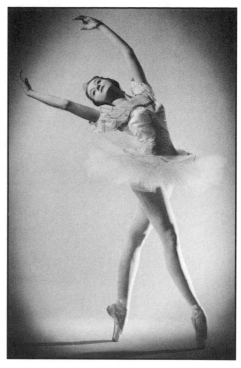

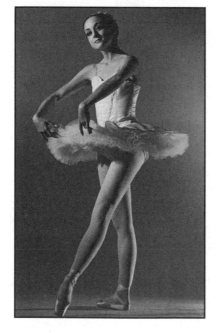

"Some of my favorite ballet roles were La Coquette in *Chiarina* (above left); Raymunda in *Raymunda* (above right); and Snow Queen in *The Nutcracker* (left).

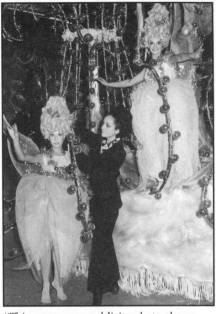

"Being a model took me from the fashion runway to television commercials and newspaper advertisements, such this national print ad."

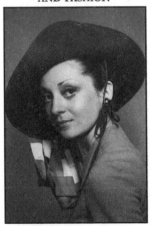

"This newspaper publicity photo shows me working on the Sun Bowl Parade float 'The Enchanted Forest.'"

SCHOOL OF MODELING
AND FASHION

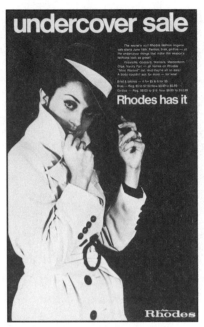

"I directed the Barbizon School of Modeling and Fashion in El Paso and then Dallas."

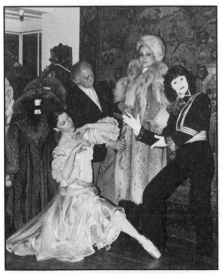

"As fashion coordinator for a San Francisco fashion extravaganza, I worked with twenty-three shops at Ghirardelli Square, a professional ballet company, and a mime troupe."

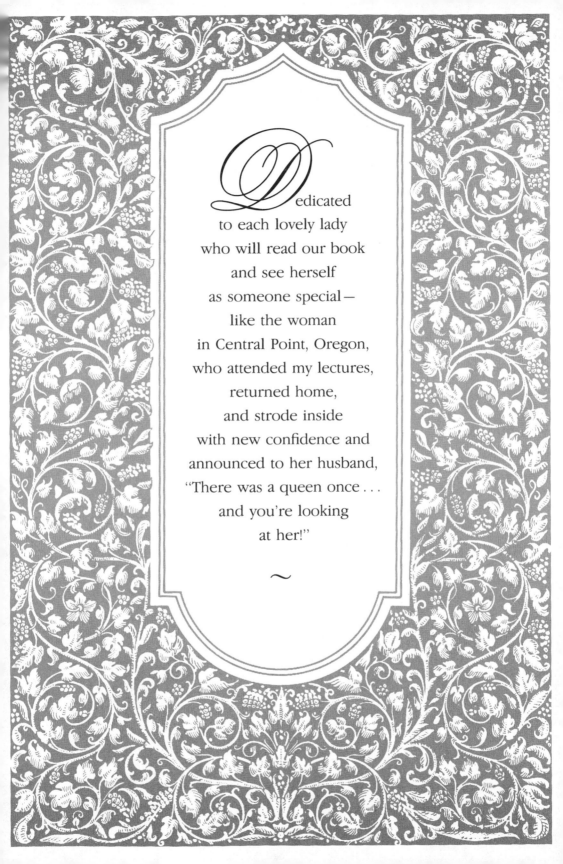

*D*edicated
to each lovely lady
who will read our book
and see herself
as someone special —
like the woman
in Central Point, Oregon,
who attended my lectures,
returned home,
and strode inside
with new confidence and
announced to her husband,
"There was a queen once . . .
and you're looking
at her!"

~

1

There Was a Queen Once . . .

*There was a queen once who reigned in troubled days. And
every time the country was on the brink of war and the people
were ready to fly into a panic, she would put on her showiest
dress and most cheerful manner and move graciously among
them. When the people saw the queen riding by, they were convinced that all was well — and thus she tided over many a danger.*

This is the beginning of a much longer fable I related to a
group of women in a conference at Chehalis, Washington, in
March 1988. At the time I was unaware of the dramatic impact
the story would have in the life of one member of my audience.
That person, Cindy Wilson, and I had never met.

The parable describes a young couple, John and Jennie Mungrave, who eagerly fell in love, married, and bought a farm, but
found joy slipping away from them as the years passed by. John
worked late into the night, and Jennie took more and more of
the backbreaking physical tasks upon her own shoulders, desperately attempting to help her husband, but in the process losing
herself.

One hot afternoon Jennie was lifting heavy baskets of tomatoes
when a beautiful, stylishly dressed stranger stopped to purchase
some apples. Obviously a woman of quality, the stranger was no
longer young, but Jennie envied the aura of youth and hope that
clung to her. In turn, the stranger saw a woman who was still
young but haggard and weary, eyes hard and listless, her calico
dress shapeless and begrimed. The woman's attitude invited shar-

ing, and before she could stop herself, Jennie poured out her troubles, describing how difficult life was and how on this very day Henry Davis was coming to foreclose on their mortgage.

When Jennie had finished talking, the woman gently told her about the queen. "And I've tried to be like her." she said. "Whenever a crisis comes in my husband's business, or when he's discouraged, I put on my prettiest dress and prepare the best dinner I can make. And somehow it works."

As Jennie watched the erect figure disappear down the lane, she wondered to herself, "Suppose . . . suppose . . . suppose . . ." So Jennie brushed her hair, changed her shoes, and put on her one good dress. Then, with something of the burning zeal of a fanatic, she attacked the confusion in the kitchen. When everything was in order, she began planning for supper. She decided to prepare fried ham, browned potatoes, apple sauce, and hot biscuits. And pie. With a spirit of daring recklessness, she spread her only white cloth on the table.

Cold fear struck Jennie's heart when Mr. Davis's car came up the drive, but again she heard the stranger's calming words: "There was a queen once . . ."

She welcomed Mr. Davis warmly and invited him in. When he hesitated, Jennie smiled warmly, in spite of the pounding of her heart, and said, "You've never tasted my hot biscuits with butter and honey, or you wouldn't take so much coaxin'!"

When John opened the kitchen door, he stared at the scene before him. Judging by the extra plate, Mr. Davis was staying for supper. Their guest grew more congenial as he ate, and so did John. Finally Mr. Davis, convinced that the lives of the Mungraves had taken a turn for the better and that his investment was secure, extended their mortgage for the next two years.

A wave of color swept up in Jennie's sallow cheeks. John looked more grateful tonight than he had for some time. Maybe he needed something else from her, even more urgently than he needed her backbreaking work.

"There was a queen once . . ."

Cindy Wilson sat motionless in her seat in the chapel in Chehalis, Washington. The example of the queen had touched a spot deep within her soul. There were similarities to Jennie's life in her own circumstances.

Cindy thought of the seventy-acre farm she helped her husband to run, with all of its accompanying demands, and how the needs of her five lively children filled every other available moment. She sighed, picturing the mountains of work that waited for her.

She had felt like a wallflower all her life, and since their last baby, she had tipped the scales at 266 pounds. Carrying around that much weight, she was always exhausted. Though time was precious, she indulged in three-hour naps. She loved hot popcorn dripping with butter, and doted on candy-covered licorice. She had never worn makeup nor seriously tried to make herself attractive; actually, she had had no idea where to begin.

She and her husband were very poor, with not even two spare dimes to jingle in their pockets. A fire had left them destitute. But then, like Jennie Mungrave in the story, she remembered the queen and dared to wonder, "Suppose . . . suppose . . . suppose . . ."

Although effecting change is one of the most difficult challenges of the human experience, at that moment Cindy gave herself permission to change. Maybe she didn't look like a queen — not yet — but she could feel like one inside. Unbeknownst to me, she had taken notes like crazy. (She was armed with dozens of helps you'll learn later in this book.) I'd quoted a favorite saying of Sharlene Wells, Miss America 1985 — "Fake it till you make it!" — and that was exactly what Cindy resolved to do.

Time passed. It was now August 1990. I was in Provo, Utah, in the middle of teaching a session at Brigham Young University Education Week when a pretty, slender woman approached me and said, "I have something to say. May I use the microphone?" A little hesitant, I agreed.

"My name is Cindy Wilson," she began. I could tell she was

nervous. I put my arm around her shoulders to steady her and felt her body shaking like a leaf.

"I've always had a weight problem, but after my last baby I weighed 266 pounds," she confessed. "I lost down to 232 and thought, 'Well, I guess I'm going to be stuck there for the rest of my life.'" This was greeted with sympathetic chuckling from the audience, as if they understood.

"Then Barbara came to our stake women's conference," she continued. "I played my violin. And I was so inspired by everything she taught that I started wearing a little makeup. I exercised. I stopped eating sugar—even added some color to my hair. I'm still struggling, but I've gained much more confidence. I thought I should let Barbara know that and publicly thank her."

I couldn't help breaking in. "How much weight have you lost now?"

Cindy's face lit up as she exclaimed, "Over one hundred pounds!" She was followed by thunderous applause as she returned to her seat.

There had to be more to the story. I took her name and phone number, and a few months later I called her and said, "I know you'll think this is weird, but would you allow me to fly you to my home in California? I'd like to know more about you."

When she arrived, we perched on the bed in our guest room, even before she unpacked, and she filled me in on her life. Here is what she said, in her own words:

"My husband and I bought a dairy farm, complete with a house that was one hundred years old. Our neighbor wanted to sell his old house, same ancient vintage, but we liked it a lot. We bought it and moved it to our property, intending to fix it up, live in it, and rent out our own house to help meet the payments. We weren't worried when the insurance company wouldn't insure it until renovation was complete.

"Then one Sunday afternoon the house we'd just bought went up in flames. Burned to the ground. With no insurance. For months we were tied to double payments—for our farm and for the house that was only a memory. It didn't help when we lost our entire corn crop in a killer windstorm.

"We paid off the house on January 1, 1990, and breathed a sigh of relief. Then, on January 9, our area suffered the worst flood in Washington's history, and we were directly in its path. Two rivers rose and met and raced through our barn, sweeping away our bales of hay. The current crashed through our house while I frantically emptied cupboards, stacking supplies on the couch until their weight broke that down. Our freezer turned upside down and floated off down the river, bobbing like a child's toy, and so did our cases of food storage. Having passed through the barn, the water dropped a gooey, yellowish silt with a horrendous smell.

"When the floodwaters finally receded, everything we owned was either missing or in shambles. Even the clothes in the closets were not fit to wear. Our wooden floors still buckle. I'm not sure when we can afford to replace them."

Cindy opened her suitcase. "Before you see them," she said, "I should tell you that all the clothes I have now I got from the Salvation Army." What I saw was that using the fashion tips she learned in my seminars and with her ability to sew, she had put together several extraordinarily effective outfits. One aqua suit had been a size twenty before she cut it down to half that size. It was lovely. She could have worn it anywhere.

All of us encounter rough spots. What matters is, do we get ourselves past them, or do we trip and fall flat on our face? I'm sure by now you're wondering what Cindy did to change, so here it is.

Cindy chose to keep her focus on the Savior. She and her family studied the scriptures together and held family home evenings regularly. Her attitude changed from blind obedience to knowledgeable independence. Now she understands what she believes.

Still sitting on our bed, Cindy explained, "You said to go out and buy a beautiful crystal goblet, just for me, to make myself start to feel like a queen. You said to buy a bud vase and keep

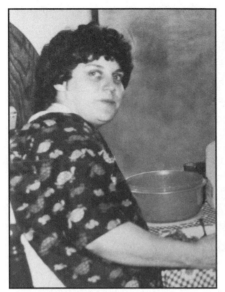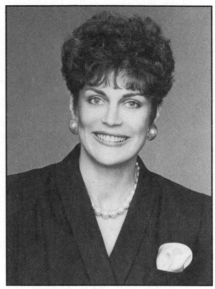

Cindy Wilson before and after she lost weight and changed her image

fresh flowers in it, and a special place mat for regal lunches, so I splurged. I used and savored these treasures, and sure enough, I began to feel queenly.

"In the conference you said to start exercising, so I enrolled in a tap-dancing class and swallowed hard when my husband teased me, calling me his 'two-ton tapper with the thunder thighs.' But tap dancing didn't work. I developed blisters on my inner thighs to the point that it hurt me to walk."

Then, Cindy said, she remembered a story I had told at the conference in Chehalis about a woman who started to lose weight by running to her mailbox and back. The woman gradually increased the distance until she was running for forty-five minutes each day, six days a week. "I followed her example and did it, too," Cindy said. "At first my husband was embarrassed. Everything jiggled. But I found that exercise gave me energy. In addition, you'd said simply to cut out sugar, fat, and salt, and to eat things the way God made them. I remembered you saying he doesn't caramelize apples on the tree, and you don't cut open a fresh potato and find it filled with bacon bits."

She watched the scales and learned to love the figure 9—
259, 229, 189. Each descent into the next group of ten was a
victory.

"Not long ago, I thought I deserved a treat," she concluded.
"I'd popped one licorice candy into my mouth when my son
snatched the others out of my hand and ran out the door. He
couldn't stand to see me eat them. That made me realize how
proud my whole family is of me and how they support me in my
endeavor to change. My husband isn't embarrassed or laughing
anymore."

Yes, "There was a queen once..."

...and *this* queen's name is Cindy.

Maybe you'd be interested in how another queen was born.
Jean Joseph was a shy sixth-grader on the day when something
inside her shriveled up and died. On that day, she read the
inscription in her school yearbook, scrawled across the entire
back page: "To the Ugliest Girl in Centerville." The inscription
was written by a boy, so of course it had to be true.

Did the author of the phrase mean to scar his classmate for
life? No, of course he didn't. No one would deliberately be that
cruel. The boy was young and immature, and undoubtedly he
meant the cut as a joke. But for Jean, at that vulnerable age when
she was sorting out exactly who and what she was, the experience
was confirmation that in this game called life, she had nothing
worthwhile to give.

Jean says, "I was born and raised in the Church and have
always been active. I attended Ricks College, served a mission,
married in the temple, and have two beautiful children. Yet with
all my activity, and though my testimony of the gospel was strong,
I suffered from a debilitating lack of self-confidence.

"I knew I was ugly; it was down in writing. I was always one
of the tallest in my class, and that made me more self-conscious.
In speech class I didn't like the way I spoke, so I didn't open my
mouth if I could help it. I hated going to social events because
I always felt sick there. If I had to go, I drove my own car so I
wouldn't feel trapped. The more I retreated into myself, the

more that hurtful yearbook quotation became a self-fulfilling prophecy."

Isn't it interesting how often physical ailments follow ailments of the spirit? Over a period of twelve years Jean underwent numerous major, painful, and frightening surgeries, which added to her dejection.

In January 1986, I spoke to wives at an overnight scout excursion, while their husbands were occupied elsewhere. I didn't know Jean at the time. She didn't want to go to the outing, she says, and she cried all through my lecture on building self-esteem. Some of the examples hit too close to home.

After my talk, Jean hid in the rest room and cried some more. But through her tears she felt a faint glimmer of hope. Was it possible — could even she feel better about herself if she worked at it? She scanned notes from my class and analyzed her situation. Her spiritual side seemed to be in order, but clearly something else was lacking.

Jean lives close enough to me that we could visit, and I was genuinely interested in her. We talked about the importance of color in building one's confidence, and since she was concerned about weight, we discussed methods of bringing that under control. (She was the woman I'd spoken of who began her exercise program by running to the mailbox and back.)

I took Jean to my hair stylist for a new, more attractive cut for her face and personality, and to a makeup expert. Jean has beautiful eyes, and she learned how to apply mascara and subtle shadow to draw out their beauty.

As her confidence increased, not in giant leaps but by inches, she enrolled in college and studied to be a fashion designer. I knew how much her self-esteem had grown when she came right out and admitted to me that she got straight A's. But change is seldom easy. Jean went through a period when her health became worse again, and the medicine she needed had disastrous side effects. She rapidly gained eight pounds but lost them again. Then colitis struck, and she gained another eight pounds in two days, accompanied by a painful rash.

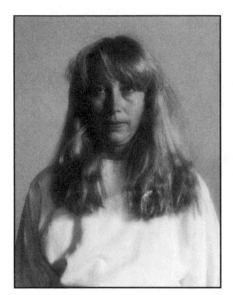 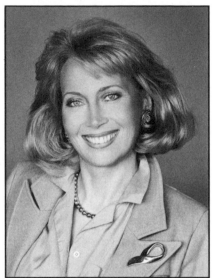

Jean Joseph: from "The Ugliest Girl in Centerville" to a confident woman

Jean says, "When my legs swelled up like balloons, I clung to everything I had learned about the philosophy of internal strength, and to prayer. Realizing I had reached some of my goals, I determined not to give up. If that level of pain and suffering had accosted me a few years ago, I believe I would have given in and died. But not now. I had come too far to let it go."

Jean was in tune with the Spirit, and also tuned in to service. As her health improved, she studied to be a color consultant. She wanted to give to others what she herself had received, and since one of the side effects of service is that it blesses the life of the giver, her knowledge of color spilled over and splashed throughout her home. Jean responds best to light colors, but her house had been dark. With the small amounts of money she earned as a color consultant, and with the skill at decorating she learned in college, she started buying furniture to lighten and enhance her home. Nowadays it is a lovely and peaceful spot.

Jean didn't change her personality to another one that wasn't right for her. Instead she worked hard to improve what she basically was. She is quiet still, but with a poised and attractive serenity. She has the regal stance of a queen. And today, as this book is being written, she is serving as the Relief Society president in her ward.

Jean explains, "I shudder when I look back at my life before I took control. Nobody should have to live with such constricting doubts and fears. Losing weight and learning to be more attractive on the outside were only means to an end, but they were what I needed to set my spirit free.

"Now, a few years and lots of hard work later, I wear a size eight. But the important thing is that when I look in the mirror today, I smile at the real me and she smiles back."

I echo the importance of what Jean said. Like yourself. Think of yourself as a queen. You are a daughter of God. Work toward the day when you too can smile at yourself in a mirror, and the real you will smile back.

2

My "Winner's Formula"

The first time I stood in a room filled with contestants for the crown of Miss USA, I looked around and my heart sank. The woman I had coached was gorgeous, but they were all gorgeous. Every one. Seeing that many beautiful women in one spot is an awe-inspiring experience.

I looked more closely. From the standpoint of beauty alone, any one of the entrants could win. What would be the deciding factor? Beauty alone wouldn't do it. That was obvious. The winner needed an edge, something special. From that moment on, I began to develop what I now call my "Winner's Formula."

Exerting the power to change anything that we have become accustomed to is probably the hardest thing we ever attempt. Change, even change for the better, seems to go against human nature. Kris Mackay wrote a magazine article about a marvelous, lifesaving invention, a solar cook box conceived by two grandmothers in Arizona, which is now being introduced to third-world countries around the globe. The cooker can be put together out of scrap materials. It isn't expensive. It isn't high-tech. It's so simple to make and so easy to use that the prospect for changing or even saving lives boggles the imagination.

Dr. Robert Metcalf, a microbiology professor at California State University at Sacramento, is one of the dedicated people who are volunteering their time and efforts to trying to upgrade the health and nutrition of people in far-flung places where deforestation and polluted water are rampant. One of the keys to this program is the simple solar cook box.

13

How was the box initially received? Dr. Metcalf tells about standing in a tiny cooking hut in Bolivia and being almost blinded by acrid smoke from the fire of twigs that an exhausted woman had trudged miles that day to gather. He watched as she stirred her pot, tears coursing down her cheeks from the sting of the smoke. He had brought with him a gift—the solar cook box—that would let her leave the hut and cook her family's meals in comfort in the open air. All she had to do was agree to change.

Incredibly, her first response was, "If this *gringo* thinks he can cook with the sun, he's got to be crazy!" Now the project is going very well, but it is a miracle the professor did not become discouraged and quit before the box was given a chance.

Willingness to change is the key ingredient in any program for improvement. To insure that the young women I was coaching for the Miss USA competition would stand out beyond the others like the proverbial beacon on a hill, to give them that noticeable edge, I decided their approach should be altered. They must be willing to work for more than just beauty. Together we would change toward a whole and balanced package.

After considerable thought, I concluded that there are four basic facets to personality, and that these four facets are each essential for any individual to be well-rounded and whole. Thus, they comprise my winner's formula: *Mental, Physical, Spiritual, and Social.*

This formula is one that the Savior Himself exemplified, for in the scriptures we learn that "Jesus increased in wisdom [mental] and stature [physical], and in favor with God [spiritual] and man [social]." (Luke 2:52.)

Figure 1 (page 15) illustrates how the winner's formula works. The triangle illustrates the mental, physical, and spiritual components of our lives. Each of these components is involved with self—*my* mental self; *my* physical self; *my* relationship with Deity—and each should be developed in order to give balance to the other sides. The circle inside the triangle stands for the social part of the formula, our interaction with our fellow beings.

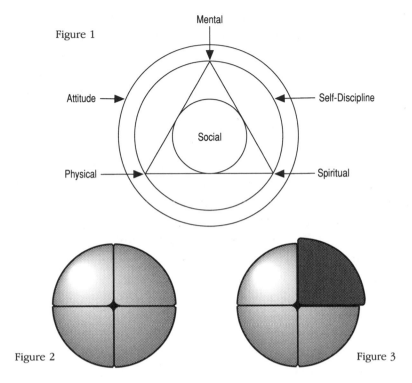

Figure 1

Mental

Attitude → ← Self-Discipline

Social

Physical — ← Spiritual

Figure 2   Figure 3

This aspect is developed as we go outside of ourselves and forget ourselves in service to others.

The outer circles surrounding the four aspects of the formula represent *attitude and self-discipline,* two vital keys to successful accomplishment. As we develop good habits through attitude and self-discipline, each day those habits become ingrained in us and more difficult to break.

Another way to visualize this concept is to think of a ball divided into four quarters. (See figure 2.) If each quarter is balanced equally, the ball will bounce and return in a predictable manner. If one quarter is developed unnaturally or looms considerably larger than the other three, who knows where the ball will ricochet? (See figure 3.) Strengthening the weak quarters should bring the ball back into balance.

Look now at the four components of the winner's formula.

Which ones are the strongest for you? Which one do you need to build up in order to have more balance in your life?

My husband believes that each of us is born with at least one side out of our four that is stronger. We find one area easier to work on and more fun than the others. Mine is physical. That's why I ended up as a dancer. I enjoy doing physical things. I love to exercise. I don't particularly like to read. When I should be bolstering my mental capacity, I tell myself I can't because there are closets to organize or floors to mop. I find enjoyment in all the physical self-disciplines. But I'm trying. Taped to my mirror is this cryptic message: "Read a book!"

And that balance, that inner glow which comes from trusting in the goodness of the Lord, that feeling of confidence as a result of mental and physical self-discipline, that inner beauty fostered by committing ourselves to the righteous service of others — each of these is, I am convinced, what made titled queens out of so many of the young women I helped to train.

A good illustration of how to apply the winner's formula is a young woman I met in October 1990, while visiting in Salt Lake City. Elizabeth Johnson called me, introduced herself, and asked for my help. "I'm planning to be in the Miss Utah pageant," she said, "but I have some real problems." Now, I have a very busy schedule, and it is impossible for me to work personally with every young woman who calls me seeking training for a beauty pageant. If she is not already a state winner, I am forced to tell her that I simply don't have the time. But I agreed to meet briefly with Elizabeth, thinking that I couldn't take her on as a client, but maybe I could give her some pointers. This is the story she told me.

Elizabeth had participated in the Miss Utah pageant the year before and had been thrilled to be chosen as second runner-up. Her talent as a concert pianist helped boost her to that spot. Surely, she told herself, next year she could win. She had purchased my *Inside, Outside Beauty Book* and had studied my winner's formula. (She had even laminated some of the book's pages.)

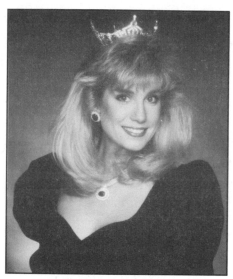

Elizabeth Johnson, Miss Utah 1992

Shortly after the pageant was over, she was driving on a freeway when her car stalled. She needed to push it to the side of the road, so she got out and held the door open with her left hand while she reached inside to steer with her right.

Suddenly she noticed another car bearing down on her, and it was coming fast. It sped closer and closer. Helplessly she watched it come, powerless to stop it or to get out of the way. She couldn't believe it would hit her, but it did, breaking both of her legs and mashing her left hand against her car's door, severing most of the nerves. Her right hand was also severely damaged when it crashed through the windshield. In the hospital later, swathed in bandages and casts, she was devastated when doctors told her she would never play the piano again.

Elizabeth was furious with her Heavenly Father. How could He do this to her, taking away the talent she had worked all her life to develop? Bitterness toward Him splashed over onto her attitude toward her family, and she became difficult to live with.

One day, sitting in her wheelchair in the hospital, Elizabeth was approached by a sweet little girl who asked, "Do you play the piano?" Elizabeth answered bitterly, through clenched teeth,

"Well, I used to." The little girl pulled her hands from behind her back. Her fingers were twisted and misshapen, but a smile lit up her face. "My daddy says I won't ever be able to play the piano," she said, "but that God gave me ears so I can enjoy listening when somebody else plays."

As she recuperated, Elizabeth made up her mind that having once been an accomplished pianist, she would regain her skills on her own, no matter what the cost. She forced her hands to play the piano. With no feeling at all in the fingers of her left hand, she trained herself to feel through her palm.

The doctor warned her not to use her legs until they were completely healed. He even added weights to the casts so she wouldn't be tempted. But again she gritted her teeth, and she stubbornly walked on her treadmill. At her next examination, he was horrified. "What have you done to yourself? The fractures are not healing. In fact, they are worse."

The bandages and casts were gone when I met Elizabeth. And because of what she had been through, I agreed to make time to work with her. The first time she came to my home in California, I questioned her about how she was doing with the four points in my winning formula. Mental? An honor student in accelerated classes. Physical? She was now working out an hour every day. Spiritual? She was president of her Laurel class in the Young Women program, and she read the scriptures daily.

Elizabeth was surprised when I said, "You're doing well in so many things. Even so, it's really too bad you're not going to win. You've turned so deeply into yourself—saying *my* mind, *my* body, *my* spirituality—that you've missed the whole concept of service to others, the main quality a winner should have. You're doing nothing for anybody but Elizabeth."

My husband, Hal, gave her a blessing and told her to reach out to others and to be a light to her family. She felt the Spirit and went home with new resolve, and we continued to work together.

Two weeks before the pageant, Elizabeth came back to my home. She had followed all my advice and trained intensely, trying hard to get out of herself in the process. Yet something was still missing. This time I told her, "Elizabeth, the way you will win this pageant is to forget yourself and focus on the Savior. Surrender all you are or can be to Him. That is the most important advice of all."

She went home and continued to work on preparing herself. I sent her a large picture of the Savior, identical to the one she had seen in my home. She took that picture with her to the Miss Utah pageant and placed it backstage so she could see it while she competed. She prayed, "Heavenly Father, I want to serve a mission for you. Let me know your desires. If this is my mission, please show me. If it isn't, I will talk to my bishop about a regular mission tomorrow." She ended her prayer, "When I go out on stage, will you walk with me?" Then she heard the still, small voice say, "Elizabeth, I will not only walk with you, I will escort you."

I was not able to be there the night of the pageant finals, so Elizabeth's mother carried a portable phone and called me from the auditorium with the results. When I answered, I could hear the applause. Her first words to me were, "She's walking the ramp!" Elizabeth had been crowned Miss Utah!

Someone once said that if a woman isn't beautiful at twenty, it isn't her fault; but if she isn't beautiful at forty-five, she has only herself to blame. Have you noticed how some people age unattractively while others grow old looking like angels — or queens?

Janice Kapp Perry wrote a beautiful song, "The Woman You'll Be Someday," that provides a fitting conclusion to this discussion:

I see an old woman rocking there,
The sun shining softly on her silver hair.
I wonder the secrets she holds deep inside,
Is she smiling or hiding a tear in her eye?
She watches our day as her story unfolds,
For you see, she is you, grown old.
And with every decision you make today,
You're creating the woman you'll be someday.
Just for now the old woman depends on you.

She waits and she watches
As you make her dreams come true.
Be kind to the woman waiting there,
For time passes swiftly and you must prepare. . . .
Be watchful, young woman, choose well today!
Remember to live for the woman you'll be someday.

I am convinced that when we follow the winning formula—when we are well balanced and developed mentally, physically, spiritually, and socially—and when our focus is on the Savior, we can, as Hal likes to say, carry the glow of knowing that we are "right with God."

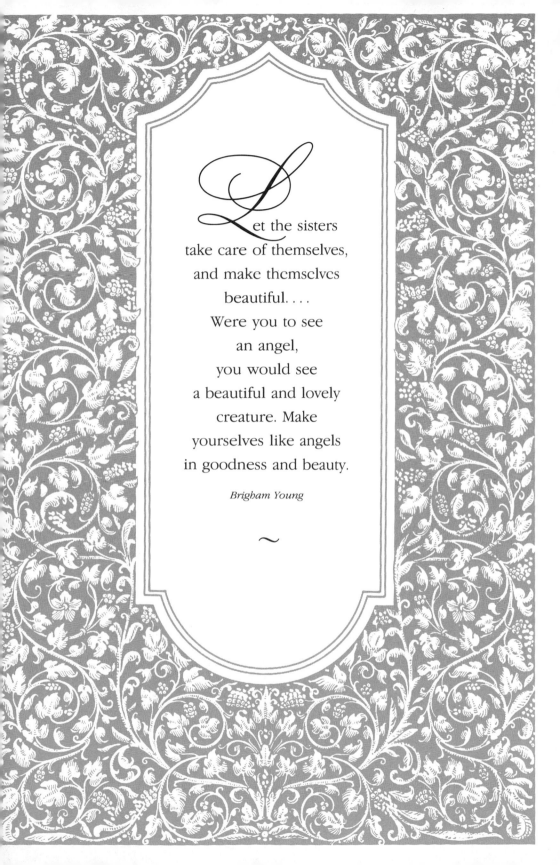

*L*et the sisters
take care of themselves,
and make themselves
beautiful. . . .
Were you to see
an angel,
you would see
a beautiful and lovely
creature. Make
yourselves like angels
in goodness and beauty.

Brigham Young

~

3

Portraying Grace and Beauty

In chapter 1, I talked about making ourselves into queenly women—women whose interior and exterior beauty will last through the eternities. A dictionary definition of a queen is "a woman noted for her beauty or accomplishments." But I believe that definition can be expanded. In her book *The Bible's Legacy for Womanhood,* author Edith Dean refers to queenly beauty in this way:

"Beauty took in much then [in biblical times] as now, magnetism, a natural dignity, good judgment, courteous manners, tenderness, thoughtfulness, poise, serenity, kindness, love, and an undefinable radiance, like a light within. These qualities seem to proclaim what Washington Irving has called a divinity within that makes the divinity without. Such a woman enables others who come into her presence to remember that she has a God who is great enough to believe and rely upon."

Brigham Young, the great Mormon prophet and colonizer, also referred to this kind of queenly beauty. He said, "Beauty must be sought in the expression of the countenance, combined with neatness and cleanliness and graceful manners."

To me, this means the elegance, the poise, and the beauty needed to be a queen. In this chapter, I'd like to share with you some of my ideas about how you can work on the physical you, a concern not only of beauty queens, but also of each woman who wants to look and feel her best so that this facet of the formula will be as balanced as the other three.

Serious self-improvement requires dedication and discipline and a lifetime commitment to change. Does this sound hard? Not if you take it step by step until you form good habits that will lead to the changes you want to make.

My husband's mother had a wonderful illustration on the subject of habit-forming. Suppose you take a single string and stretch it to the breaking point. It breaks. Now suppose you take seven strings, a week's worth. A little harder to break, but not impossible. But then suppose you take 365 strings, one for each day of the year, and put them together. What do you have? A rope, and a rope doesn't break. (Keep in mind that this illustration applies not only to good habits but also to bad ones.)

Some changes will take time. You can't lose all the weight you might want to lose overnight—that takes time. But there are some things you can do right now, to bring results instantly. From this moment on, you can start being a more confident you. Let's begin.

1. Improve Your Posture

Stand tall. The scriptures tell us that we are of "royal birth," so pretend that you are a member of royalty and that three strings are attached to your head—one at the crown and one on each ear. Make believe an angel is pulling the strings gently, pulling your entire body upward toward heaven in perfect alignment, lifting you straight up out of your shoes. Your neck becomes longer and swanlike, eliminating much of the sag women tend to develop there. (Be certain your string lifts you from the crown or back of the top of your head, not the forehead, where your chin will be lifted and you will appear snooty.)

At the same time, pull your stomach not only in but up, into your chest. This is the most important element of good posture.

With exaggerated motions, roll your shoulders forward, then push them up toward your ears, then way back, and finally down. This will make your head and neck high, your shoulders back and down. (By this time your stomach will have popped out again, so pull it again up into your chest.)

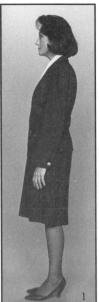 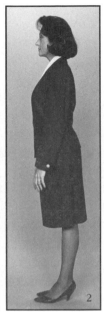 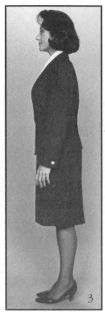 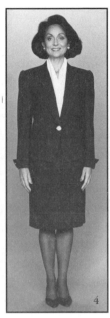 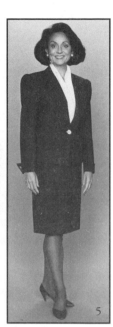

(1) Poor posture—shoulders slumped, stomach protruding. (2) Poor posture—posterior protruding. (3) Improved posture—standing tall, shoulders back, stomach in and up. (4) Good posture helps project confidence. (5) The stance that makes you look ten pounds thinner.

I can hear you say, "I look better, but that position doesn't feel comfortable." It won't for a while, but just keep at it. Natural is not necessarily desirable. Babies are not born with acceptable behavior in all things; they have to be trained. Echoing that philosophy, my husband, Hal, who is a successful business executive, says, "Sometimes we have to do what we don't want to do in order to get what we want to get." (See photos 1–4.)

2. Take a Queenly Stance

Do you want to look ten pounds thinner in a photograph—instantly? Try taking the basic model's stance. Here's how. Put both feet together. Position your toes so they are pointing to 12 o'clock on the face of an imaginary clock. Next, leaving the right foot in place, slide the left foot back so that the heel of the right foot is in the center or arch of the left foot and the left toe is pointing to 10 o'clock. Flex your knees slightly, and rest most of your body weight on the back (left) foot. Now turn your body in the direction of the left foot, then turn your head to face the camera. *Voila!* Ten pounds thinner. (See photo 5.)

If it feels more comfortable, you can reverse the position of your feet and put the right foot behind the left. Just imagine facing 12 o'clock and slide the right foot back so that the toe is pointing to 2 o'clock, and the heel of the left foot is in the arch of the right foot. Then turn your body in the direction of the right foot, and turn your head to face the camera.

Another tip: As you take this stance, allow your arms to fall gracefully, covering the outline of each hip. Don't clench your fists or bend your elbows. Let your fingers and arms hang long and gracefully like those of a ballerina. That will help hide curves or extra silhouette bulges.

This stance is not just for photographs. Use it whenever you can to make yourself look more graceful, poised, queenly. It will make a difference. Don't imagine people are saying, "Oh, my! What is she doing with her feet?" No one will notice; they will just see an air of elegance.

3. Establish Eye Contact

Never look at the ground, whether you are communicating with someone in person or through the camera. In any competition, a judge loses confidence in the contestant who periodically looks at the ground. It makes her appear self-conscious. Look people (or the camera) in the eye. Look interested. Smile. Christina Faust, Miss California 1989, is a master at exhibiting genuine interest in face-to-face contact. She never shakes hands with just one hand. She reaches out with both hands to encircle the hand she shakes. It is a small gesture, perhaps, but one that exudes warmth and produces instant friendships.

4. Walk Like a Queen

The movements of a confident woman should be simple, natural, and smooth. Her arms should hang naturally from the shoulder, with the inside of each arm turned toward her body.

Each arm swings slightly, approximately eight inches forward and backward. To make the movement smooth while you are walking, imagine that you are floating on a cloud. When you go up or down stairs, give the impression that you are gliding by trailing your fingers lightly on the bannister. This will also help you with balance.

A happy walker moves quickly and is light on her feet. A dejected walker shuffles along, hands in pockets, not knowing or caring where she is headed.

The confident woman maintains a happy walk regardless of how she feels inside. Her walk gives the impression that she is confident and that all is well even though that may be an illusion at the moment.

Throughout my years of ballet training, I learned how to use my body to illustrate a character. I learned to move like an old person, an angry person, even an insane person, as in the mad scene in the ballet *Giselle*. I've often thought that because dancers learn so much about the body and how it looks when it's older, they know which postures to avoid as they themselves age.

5. Sit and Rise Gracefully

No matter how gracefully you enter a room, all is lost if you plop into a chair or sofa.

Position yourself in front of a chair in the basic model's stance. Feel the chair against the calf of your back leg. Imagining that three strings on the top of your head are being pulled gently, lower your body straight down to the edge of the chair. Touch your hands to the chair lightly for positioning; then slide back into place, leaving your back still erect.

Repeat the process in reverse when getting up. First, slide to the chair's edge. Now rise, using the muscles of your thighs to lift yourself gracefully. Don't hoist yourself up awkwardly by pushing on the chair or grasping another object for support.

When you are sitting, assume a position that looks graceful. Be sure you keep your knees together. Here are five positions that work well:

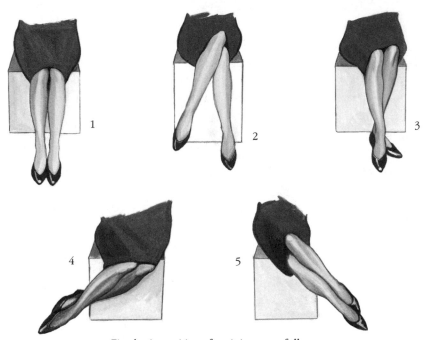

Five basic positions for sitting gracefully

1. Place both feet on the floor, with your toes pointing straight ahead.

2. Starting with both feet on the floor, toes pointing straight ahead, cross one leg over the other at the knee. This is the most basic sitting position.

3. Position your feet in the basic model's stance.

4. Gently swing both feet to one side or the other and cross your ankles.

5. Gently swing one foot to one side (it doesn't matter which side) and cross the other leg over at the knee so that your legs and feet together make one graceful line. This is an especially graceful position if you have long legs.

The way in which you hold your hands while sitting can also affect your appearance. The basic positions are (1) with both palms up; (2) with both palms down; (3) with one palm up and one down; or (4) with your fingers lightly laced. (See illustrations, page 29.)

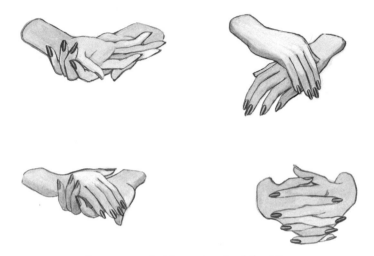

Four ways to hold your hands while sitting

Any of these combined hand and leg positions creates an attractive picture in everyday life, whether you are sitting in your own living room with a guest or being interviewed for a job. Sit in front of a mirror and practice the combination that feels most comfortable and looks most graceful for you.

6. Wear Colors That Flatter You

I am convinced that color is one of the most effective instant beauty aids available. Colors are magic. Colors have power. Wearing your most flattering colors can help make you look younger, more vital, and rested. And wearing colors that are not flattering can make you look older, run-down, and tired.

Colors can also affect your opinions and impressions of others. When you first meet a woman, you probably (if you're like most people) notice her face, then the rest of her body. Whether you realize it or not, the colors she wears make an impression on you, even before you greet her or shake her hand. If she is wearing colors that are flattering to her, you will form a positive impression that says, "This person looks great."

To gain more self-confidence and always look your best, try to find out which shades are better for you and which ones to avoid. Fortunately, unraveling the mystery of color is not complicated.

One way I recommend to determine color selection is the seasonal color theory, which is based upon the colors found in nature during each of the seasons. Entire books have been written on this theory, but in essence, this is what it says: *Winter* is characterized by the vivid primary colors — red, yellow, and blue — and sharp contrasts of black and white. *Spring* bursts forth with bright shades of yellows and greens, such as chartreuse. *Summer* emerges in muted shades such as pastel blues and pinks. *Autumn* unfolds with rich, warm, earthen hues of golds and browns.

Sometimes women have told me they were informed that they are 10 percent "winter," 15 percent "spring," and 55 percent "fall." My response is, That's impossible!

Here is the secret, in simple terms, of how to determine what colors will enhance you. Ask yourself: Are the undertones of my skin "cool" or "warm"? How can I tell the difference? The simplest, least expensive way to find this out is to go to a large department store in your city (or the closest city, if you live in a rural or suburban area) and ask about cosmetic lines that offer both cool-shade and warm-shade cosmetics. Then ask the sales representatives to help determine whether your skin tones are cool (summer and winter seasons are cool, with an undertone of blue), or warm (spring and autumn are warm, with an undertone of yellow or gold).

If your skin tones are cool, here are colors that should enhance your skin tones:

Winter — pure white, pure black, charcoal gray, true red, royal blue, burgundy, dark navy.

Summer — soft white, pastel blue, pastel pink, mauve, pearl gray, rose brown, light navy.

If your skin tones are warm, here are some of your choices:

Autumn — oyster white, pumpkin, dark brown, olive green, rust, gold, camel.

Spring — ivory, apricot, bright yellow, chartreuse, peach, golden brown.

Which group of colors do you like best? Make your selection on the basis of a group of colors, not on an individual color.

To verify your choices, drape fabrics of various hues under your chin, one at a time, and examine the effect of each in a mirror. Don't concentrate on the fabric; look at your skin. Take a friend with you; she will probably see you better than you see yourself. Which colors bring life to your face and which drain you?

Your best indicator colors are silver and gold. If silver makes your face look lifeless and gray, and gold makes your skin look radiant and glowing, then you have warm undertones (spring and autumn). However, if gold makes you look jaundiced and your under-eye circles deeper, and silver makes your skin appear more flawless, then your undertones are cool (winter and summer). You may not distinguish the difference immediately, but keep trying. A pattern will emerge.

Keep in mind that your skin tone is a unique quality that will not change during your lifetime. A suntan may deepen it and age may fade it somewhat, but it will never change from one season to another. Understanding whether your coloring is cool or warm is helpful for coordination of your makeup, wardrobe, and even your hair.

Women with cool undertones should not wear makeup and clothes with golden shades; conversely, women with warm undertones *should* wear golden shades. When you use the same tones for both your makeup and your wardrobe, your entire look will be in perfect harmony.

The best rule for your hair is to keep the color as close as possible to its natural shade. As women age, they should color their hair one shade lighter rather than one shade darker. A shade that is dark can be harsh and aging. And if you highlight your hair, be sure the shade doesn't conflict with your natural color. For example, never highlight black hair with golden tones.

A Queen Needs More

These suggestions are starting points — simple, effective ways to affect your look instantly. But putting yourself together successfully can't be a matter of external beauty alone, as comforting as being attractively groomed may be. A queen needs more. Each woman must approach self-improvement as a whole, body and spirit, like a jigsaw puzzle, fitting in with equal care the pieces of external beauty, internal poise, physical well-being, vibrant health, personality, and spirituality.

Some time ago my stake president issued me a calling. Knowing that I work with young women who are competing in beauty pageants, giving them help for both external and internal beauty, he wondered if the women of our stake might enjoy a similar program. He asked me if I would set aside one Saturday a month for nine months to work with sisters who were interested. He believed, as I do, that the way we feel about ourselves is reflected in the way we treat others. He expected that perhaps twenty women would sign up.

The twenty people expected to sign up for the program turned out to be a whopping seventy-five, and it was one of the most exciting experiences that I have ever had. We called the program "Metamorphosis."

The first day we took "before" pictures. The women could wear whatever they wanted. My only stipulation was that they couldn't smile. At the end of the course, we took "after" pictures.

Fifty of the women completed the course (some dropped out due to conflicts with their schedules or for other reasons). Those fifty women presented a glorious fashion show, as professional as any I have seen in New York or Los Angeles. I stood backstage and cried when I saw what they had done. If one compares their "before" and "after" pictures, it is difficult to picture them as the same women. Each one had gained much greater confidence and poise, and they were beginning to expand the scope of their lives. Some of them expressed their thoughts after completing the course:

"Being happy comes from liking yourself," said Ethel Otteson.

"You don't have to have the flawless face of a Miss USA if you have the light of Christ. You don't have to be beautiful to be 'beautiful.' Too many women are 'hiding,'" Sally Bayles commented.

Marie Pack explained, "The 'three strings' illustration taught me to pull my body into alignment after years of 'Stand up straight!' didn't. I can feel my body pull up out of the dumps."

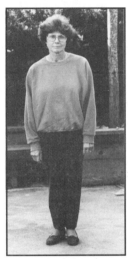 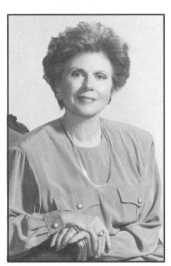

Ethel Otteson before and after "metamorphosis"

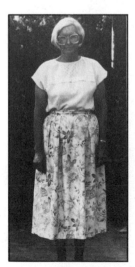 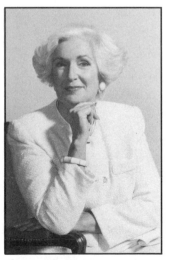

Marie Pack before and after "metamorphosis"

"After a physical, I saw my medical file at the doctor's office," Sonja Jensen reported. "I knew I was overweight, but it was a real shock to read that I was 'morbidly obese.' I went to Barbara's class with the idea that anything she could teach me I needed to learn. I'm down to 136 pounds and a size 10, and loving it. Now I know it's not selfish to spend time and money on myself. My

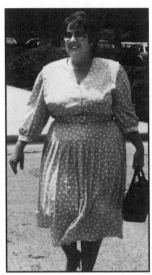 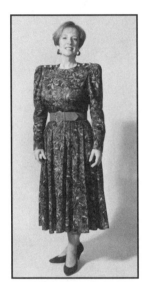

Sonja Jensen before and after "metamorphosis"

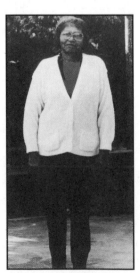 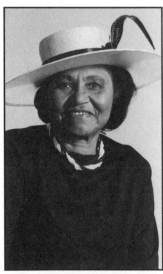

Jonnie Bell Wright before and after "metamorphosis"

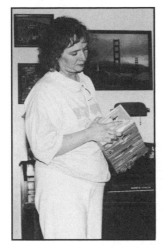 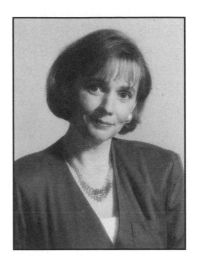

Jane Allen before and after "metamorphosis"

family appreciates much more a mom who values herself enough to look her best, rather than a frazzled, self-sacrificing martyr."

Jonnie Bell Wright believes in hands-on training. She said, "I have known women as pretty as spun silk but with hateful ways. Barbara taught us to be good Christians. You can't teach what you don't know, and you can't lead where you don't go."

Jane Allen details how added confidence enabled her to reach out for new experiences: "You have to make the best of your own circumstances and start where you are. I wanted to return to school, but it wasn't possible at the time, so I bargained with a friend. Two mornings a week, I taught her piano and she taught me Italian. She told me I have a natural ability with languages. I hadn't known that. When I began to try new things, I found I enjoyed studying tremendously.

"I was also asked to teach seminary. Teenagers had always intimidated me, and I was scared. But since I had excelled at learning Italian, I was ready to take another risk. Teaching the youth, I found I can draw on my own experiences to help others. And on vacation, I swam and even tried snorkeling. My husband said, 'Well, this is a first!' He thinks I am more fun, more exciting, and more beautiful now than when he married me. I learned in

Barbara's class that just because you are grown up, it doesn't mean you are through growing."

These women learned a most important lesson: You must be willing to try, to change what needs to be changed, even to risk a measure of failure, in order to experience success and become the most confident you possible.

4

Believe in Yourself

Some time ago I was working with a psychiatrist friend, Dr. Larry Dietz, preparing a speech for a professional women's group. Dr. Dietz asked me this question: "Barbara, who do you think has higher self-esteem — working or nonworking women?"

That was easy. I thought back several years to a political dinner I had attended with my husband, Hal, where in the course of conversation someone asked, "And what do you do?" I was sitting with people who all had careers. Wanting to fit in, I said, "I'm on the lecture circuit for Brigham Young University. I also lecture to youth, and I train young women for the Miss USA pageant."

Today I realize that if I had had more self-confidence, I would have replied, "I'm a homemaker, and I also . . . " But talking with Dr. Dietz, I blithely gave him the answer that most women give. I said that working women are more confident.

He shook his head. "No," he said. "Self-esteem is self-esteem, whether you are a working woman or not. Actually, it doesn't make any difference what you do. It's how you *feel* about yourself that counts."

Some of us are convinced that if we worked in an office, doing "important" things, instead of staying home to dust and to chauffeur the kids, our lives would be fulfilled. Still others believe that if we could slam the file drawer shut, march out of the office, and stay at home, we would never be unhappy again.

If I had a magic wand and could give you the desires of your heart, what would they be? Reach for a piece of paper, think about your circumstances, and write your wishes down. Remember, they concern you, personally. Not your husband, if you are married. Not your children. Not your parents, or nieces and nephews. On this particular list, no desire is too farfetched.

What miraculous change would make you happy? What would increase your self-esteem? What would help you feel truly contented with who you are? If you think like the majority of women I speak to, your list might look something like this:

1. Be thinner — lose weight
2. Have more education
3. Have greater spirituality
4. Have a better appearance
5. Have greater confidence, self-esteem
6. Have a more positive attitude
7. Be a better time manager
8. Have greater self-control, patience
9. Have (or develop) a talent
10. Have more money

Every item on the list represents a worthwhile goal, as does a feeling of appreciation from those whose judgment we trust. We all need strokes or accolades from family, business associates, and friends.

But the bottom line is that if you do not like yourself, if you lash out in anger, if you are prone to bitterness, frustration, or resentment, if you typically bombard others with criticism, those negative emotions are what you will receive back.

If you like yourself, however, you will automatically exhibit love, and love is exactly what you will be given in return.

Perhaps a short quiz will help pinpoint your quota of self-esteem (keep track of how many A's, B's, and C's you score).

1. How do you respond when someone says, "Wow, you're a fabulous housekeeper!"?

a. "Yes, but you should see the corners of the bathroom. They're filthy!"

b. "Oh, it's not that big a deal. I really don't put much time into it."

c. "Thank you. It's important to me to keep the house looking nice."

2. If you're furious at your husband, what do you say when he asks, "Is something wrong, honey?"
a. "Oh, nothing, dear. I'm just suffering from PMS."
b. "Well, there is this tiny little thing that's bothering me, but it's not that big a deal."
c. "Yes, there is. I'm really angry about what you said this morning. Can we talk about it?"

3. You've just got up, and you are wearing a rumpled sweatsuit, you have no makeup on, and your hair is in curlers. What do you do when your doorbell rings, and you see from the window that the woman standing there looks as if she's been up for hours?
a. You hide and hope she'll just go away.
b. You put a bag over your head and answer the door.
c. You put a cardboard McDonald's crown over your curlers, float down the stairs singing, "Here I am, Miss A-mer-ica," and open the door with a gigantic, welcoming smile. (That actually happened to me, shortly after we moved to our new home. The woman, who was from my church, nearly died laughing.)

4. You're thumbing through a fashion magazine at the doctor's office. How do you respond as you see page after page of gorgeous, pencil-thin models in the advertisements?
a. You compare yourself with every model and feel totally intimidated and unattractive.
b. You wish that you could switch places with one of those models just for a day.
c. You say to yourself, "Okay, so the models are gorgeous and pencil-thin, and they have beautiful, expensive clothes. But I love who I am. I know I have unique qualities and talents, and I wouldn't be anyone else in the world."

5. How do you respond when you look in the mirror first thing in the morning?

a. You scream and say, "Okay, that does it! I'm getting an appointment with the plastic surgeon today."

b. You wince and try to avoid looking at your reflection.

c. You stand there calmly, smile, and say to yourself, "Well, hey — I'll look *great* once I put on some makeup and fix my hair."

How did you do? If you checked mostly A's, your self-esteem needs some serious build-up. If you checked mostly B's, it could still use some help (but you're pretty average). If you checked all C's, your perception of who you are is terrific.

If you ended up with both A's and B's, how much are your feelings about yourself based on what others say about you? If television shows or magazines portray being a housewife as a lowly job, and you *are* a housewife, do you believe them? If your self-esteem is low, you accept that stereotype meekly. But if you believe in the worth of what you are doing with your life, you flatly refuse to accept that view.

Remember, self-esteem does not remain constant throughout our lives. It goes up and down like the stock market. Just when we think we have the hang of it and that our newfound confidence will go on forever, something surfaces out of nowhere, catches us off-guard, and we sink like a rock. Don't forget that with effort, our self-esteem will rise again.

We should not make unreasonable demands on ourselves for immediate perfection in all things, nor judge our self-esteem by how well we pass each test. If we do, we will be more like a yo-yo than even the stock market. The trials of some days are harder to cope with than others. Let's not let difficulties throw us.

Psychiatrists say we all need to share our frustrations. We can share them with our spouse or with another adult. A sense of humor comes in handy here, especially when examining our own shortcomings. But laughing away real weaknesses is different from unfavorably comparing ourselves with others and manufacturing weaknesses that don't exist. This is a trap even winners have to fight to avoid. I have seen contestants at the Miss USA pageant jeopardize a very real chance of winning by worrying about whether they measure up to the other contestants.

I wish I could faultlessly practice what I preach. Occasionally I get caught in the self-comparison thing too. I see how other speakers relate to young people and wonder if I'm doing all *I* can do. I want to have the same kind of influence on youth as these other speakers, because I love the young people too. But my approach is different from that of others; I can't act exactly as another speaker does because that isn't my personality. My husband, who is my best confidant, assures me, "It's like comparing a daffodil to a pine tree. You reach the kids also, but you reach them in a different way. In this life we have to use our own talents, the ones Heavenly Father gave us."

I treasure the comments in a letter to me from a woman named Mary Kelly: "So many of us need to know that we are of worth just because we are daughters of God. We need to know that He loves not only the beautiful and talented, but also the common lot of us who, though lacking in natural beauty and talent, have faith in God that He can take our dross and make it into gold. I believe that through Him, we are responsible for all of our thoughts and actions, and that the power is within us to accomplish whatever we need to change."

One facet of our personality as a whole is physical appearance. Do you like what you see in the mirror? For women especially, this is critical. If you don't like what you see, do something about it. Don't wait!

Elizabeth and Ray Murphy had a marriage she describes as "the romance of the century." Ray wrote in his life history about their meeting: "I met the sweetest girl any man could ever find. She was a beautiful, blonde nurse working at Lodgepole Hospital in Sequoia National Park. I knew she was someone special, the kind of person I had always looked for but had never found, a cut above all the other people I had ever met. And you know what? I married her! The whole world changed. And with it came a beautiful life with Liz and our children, all seven of them."

Liz describes her husband: "Ray was a tall, black-haired Irishman who was a wonderful story teller and a real Ranger [in the National Park Service]. He could shoe a horse, pack a mule, ski all day to take a snow survey, or teach rock climbing to the other Rangers. We lived in Sequoia, Yosemite, and Olympic National Parks. After our marriage, we went 'home' to a cabin at Red Fir, at 7,000 feet elevation in Sequoia. I had fun learning to cook on a wood-burning stove."

In short, life wasn't easy for Liz and Ray in terms of physical comforts or luxuries, but they had each other and their love. They enjoyed the remoteness of the forests. Their daughter Cheryl treasures memories of her parents' "one hundred honeymoons," their brief trips away, especially around October 6, their anniversary.

Ray retired in 1984 but soon was gravely ill with lymphoma. Liz was totally lost when he died just a few months later. Her doctor prescribed sleeping pills to ease her through the first endless nights, but often she stayed up late, dreading bedtime, mindlessly watching television. When she woke up after finally falling asleep, she would listen to scripture tapes to fill the long, lonely hours. Eventually she attended a few singles activities, but that didn't last; she couldn't bear to admit to herself that she was single. Fortunately, couples in her ward did not abandon her. Liz was still invited to their activities, and that was a blessing.

Liz's path crossed mine at the beginning of a class I held for women of my stake. Originally the plan had been to limit the group to fifteen women. We were ready to begin when the stake Relief Society president urged me to accept one more special sister. That was fine with me, and so Liz Murphy joined us. Thinking back, one of the highlights of the class was watching the blossoming of Liz. She changed from a woman who was lost and without purpose, having lived her entire married life in her husband's shadow, into a confident, attractive woman in her own right.

Liz says, "I'm sorry I didn't start to look better for Ray while he was still alive. But you know, he always said he saw me as young and beautiful no matter how old and fat I got. If I said,

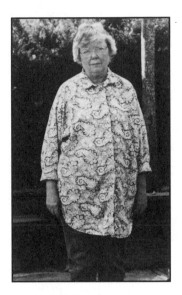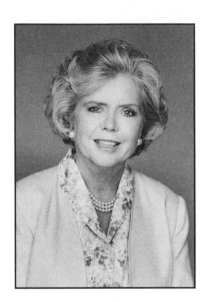

Elizabeth Murphy, who lost weight and gained greater self-confidence

'I'm a mess,' he'd say, 'Yes— a mess of loveliness.' After taking Barbara's class, I was thrilled with the difference in my self-confidence, and my children say they didn't know their mother was capable of tackling new and exciting challenges on her own.

"I believe Heavenly Father places opportunities along the paths of his children, hoping we will find the courage to reach out and help ourselves to new experiences. When the bishop asked if I'd consider a mission for the Family History Department in Salt Lake City, I'm grateful I had grown to the point of being able to accept."

As this chapter is written, Liz is serving her mission and continuing to grow.

Go back to the list of wishes you wrote down earlier. What would it take to bring them to pass? Make the changes! Don't stay in the comfortable rut you have formed for yourself. Don't wallow in the comfort of discomfort. Be like the oyster in this poem, "The Oyster and the Sand," by D. H. Elton:

> *There once was an oyster whose story I'll tell,*
> *Who found that some sand had worked under his shell.*

Just one little grain, but it gave him a pain
For oysters have feelings, for all they're so plain.

Now did he berate this working of fate
That led him to such a deplorable state?
Did he curse out the government, call for election,
And cry that the sea should have given protection?

"No!" he said to himself as he sat on the shelf.
"Since I cannot remove it, I think I'll improve it."

Well, the years rolled around as the years always do
And he came to his ultimate destiny — stew.
But the small grain of sand that had bothered him so
Was a beautiful pearl, all richly aglow.

This tale has a moral, for isn't it grand
What an oyster can do with a morsel of sand?
What couldn't we do if we'd only begin
With all of the things that get under our skin?

This poem is a lighthearted one, but it does have a moral. Make sure you like yourself. If you don't, *change*. Change means action, and action is what it takes to develop self-esteem.

5

Keeping in Tune with the Spirit

Nothing is more consistent than change. Nothing in this world lasts forever. But nobody knows better than I that in those awful, frightening moments when life hits rock bottom, it's hard to cling to faith that all will be well.

Wouldn't it be nice if the Lord would come to us, open a scrapbook of our lives, and say, "Here is what I have in store for you. Hang on just a little longer." If we could only see a photo of the wonders ahead, we would respond, "Here I am. Do with me what you will. I am in your hands."

Every day I give thanks for the present circumstances of my life. I'm married to a husband I adore, live in a beautiful, peaceful home, and have two grown children who are everything I could hope for. Today I consider myself one of the most fortunate of mortals—but it wasn't always that way.

My first marriage was to a man who suffered with severe manic depression. Remember a day when you were more depressed than at any other time, multiply that by one hundred, and you have some idea of manic depression.

We lived in Texas. One night I was onstage, dancing as the lilac fairy in *Sleeping Beauty,* when I saw him beckoning me urgently from the wings. My first thought was that something had happened to our little boy, John. I slipped offstage and he whispered, "Come with me quickly," grasping my arm and pulling me out to the car.

He threw me into the front seat, bound my wrists and ankles with adhesive tape, and gagged my mouth. Then he roared out of the parking lot and drove like a maniac for forty-five minutes. I thought he had lost his mind. When we arrived at a deserted place, he stopped the car, reached into the back seat for a shotgun, cocked it, and pointed the barrel at my leg. He said, "I'm going to destroy your knee so you will never dance again."

I have never been more terrified. I was not a Latter-day Saint at the time and had not built up a one-on-one relationship with the Lord, but with all the strength of my being I pleaded, "Heavenly Father, are you there?" For the first time in my life I heard the still, small voice. "Yes, Barbara, I'm here."

What happened next was unbelievable. My husband hesitated a moment, then uncocked the gun and drove me back to the performance hall. He pushed me — still bound and gagged — out of the car and onto the cold asphalt of the parking lot. The performance was over by then, and the lot was empty. A security guard eventually discovered me and released me from my bonds.

That was the last straw. I carried my baby over to my mother's, put him into her arms, and told her she would have to raise him. I was leaving and never coming back.

I went to Atlanta, where I continued my work with ballet and focused on my career. My mother paced the floor of her home carrying my son, while both of them cried. I didn't know she had called every church in the area, every denomination, to ask them to pray for me.

One Sunday morning I sat at the kitchen table in a house where I was boarding. From down the hall floated tinkling sounds of a music box playing "Sunrise, Sunset" from *Fiddler on the Roof.* My mind supplied the words to match the music, almost subconsciously setting the scene for how quickly children grow up. I hadn't remembered it was Mother's Day. Then I opened the newspaper and read this poem, by an unknown author:

> *"Where are you going?" you'd say to him,*
> *and "What are you going to do?"*

And with a shy smile he'd toddle outside
to slay a dragon for you.
Or perhaps there was a prince to be,
or a lion to track to its lair,
For a little boy's life is a wondrous thing,
as long as his mother's there.

"Why do birds fly all in a flock?"?
"How far are the stars from the ground?"
A thousand questions he'd ask of you;
a thousand answers you found.
"Please tell me what makes a puppy dog bark,
and why is the sky filled with air?"
Oh, a little boy's life is a learning thing,
as long as his mother's there.

"Sing me a tune," he'd say to you,
"Sing me some soft lullabies."
And you'd sit by his bed for a moment or two
until slowly he closed his eyes.
How quiet he'd be as you covered him up
and caressed his silken hair,
For a little boy's life is a peaceful thing,
as long as his mother's there.

"Don't cry," you'd say, as you held him close
when he'd fallen and hurt his head.
You held back a tear yourself, you know,
when you kissed the spot where it bled.
And the tears dried up, and the hurt went away,
under your gentle care,
For a little boy's life is a loving thing,
as long as his mother's there.

And one day you'll look up,
as the years have sped by,
And on that day it will suddenly seem to you
that he isn't a little boy anymore,
But a fine young man grown
straight and tall and true.
How fast they have gone, those childhood years,
thank God you had them to share,
For though a little boy's life is a fleeting thing,
to a mother it's always there.

I ran to the telephone and, through my tears, told my mother I was coming back for my baby. No one could ever convince me that the poem and music box combined, reaching me on that special day, were not answers to my mother's prayers and the prayers of our city's faithful who didn't even know me but were willing to beseech the Lord in my behalf.

I wish I could say that from then on my life was easy, but it wasn't. My son and I moved to Canada, but I couldn't make it alone. It was twenty degrees below zero as I took daily classes with Le Grande Ballet Canadienne, but they couldn't hire me until their European tour six months later. So my son and I stayed at a friend's apartment. I didn't even have a crib for him; he slept on a cushion on the floor, and I slept on the floor beside him.

In desperation, I went back to my husband, telling myself this time it would work. We had another baby, a little girl we named Wendy. Trying to cope with his depression, he drank more and more heavily and by now was starting to experiment with drugs.

One afternoon as I sat in the big winged-back chair in the living room, my husband's station wagon pulled into the driveway. As he walked through the front door, there was a look on his face that I had seen before. It was a look of calmness, but on the inside I knew there was a time bomb about to explode. After a few moments of trying to start an argument, he walked to my chair, grabbed me by my long hair and my arm, and dragged me up two flights of stairs and into the bathroom. He locked the door behind him and, with a determined glare and incredible strength, forced me to stand in the bathtub. He then pulled out a .44 Magnum revolver and slowly placed the barrel against my temple. With calculated calmness, he spoke slowly and deliberately: "I'm going to kill you and then kill myself." For the second time I heard the click as he cocked the trigger. I felt a rush of adrenalin, and my blood ran cold. And, for the second time, I prayed, "Heavenly Father, are you there?"

A sense of absolute calm came over me, and tears streamed down my cheeks. At that time of total need, I reached out, the Spirit responded, and we were in tune. I didn't scream or plead for my life, because I knew God was in control. (Psychiatrists tell me that calmness isn't normal behavior in such a situation. Usually women react hysterically, which often precipitates a violent response from their attacker.)

Amazingly, once again my husband uncocked the gun and my life was spared. I found out later that my grandmother had dreamed the previous night that the bodies of my husband and me were found in the bathroom, lying face down in pools of blood. Somewhat later he did take his own life.

When I met my present sweet and wise husband, Hal, one of the first things he said to me after we were well acquainted was, "Barbara, you need to get right with God." I moved to San Francisco, where we were later married, and began my intense search for truth. I started going to mass every day. Now, because of the terrifying experiences I had miraculously survived, I knew there was a God, that He lives, and that He hears and answers prayer. But as I began my study of the Bible, it was like a baby's first unsteady but exciting steps. I found myself formulating a new prayer. "Jesus Christ, who are you? Where are you?" I said that prayer every night for five years.

In 1979, after our marriage, Hal and I went on a hiking trip in another state, and our flight home took us through Salt Lake City, where we planned to stay overnight. After we were settled in a hotel, Hal suggested that we take a walk. Suddenly he said, "Look — there's the Mormon temple. Let's go inside." I was aghast. A Catholic in a Mormon temple? Hal said, "Just think of it as a historical landmark."

We wandered into the visitors' center. It seemed so foreign to my eyes. Beautiful, but bare. No candles. No crosses. No statues of saints. I thought, *These Mormons are certainly different.* Then they showed us a film, and I was more certain than ever that they were a peculiar bunch. The narrator in the film said something about a young boy who dug plates of metal out of the ground, translated them into a book (even though he didn't know the language), and conversed with angels. Strrrrange!

All at once the figure of Jesus Christ appeared on the screen.

He was dressed in white, and, with His arms outstretched, He looked directly at me, personally. In the darkness He said to me, "Barbara, here I am. Come. Follow me."

Tears flowed uncontrollably down my cheeks. "What's wrong with you?" Hal asked anxiously. I sobbed and said, "N-n-n-nothing." I wasn't ready to discuss it.

On the way out of the visitors' center we were given a card to fill out. Hal told me to write that we had enjoyed our visit but did not want them to send a representative. Being a dutiful wife, I wrote exactly that. After years of searching I had at long last found Christ, but the next move was up to Him. Surely He would not desert me now.

Two weeks later I was antiquing a piece of furniture in our garage when I noticed two clean-cut young men approaching our drive. One of them held a card in his hand, and from the way they hesitated after each step, it had to be our card saying we did not want them to come. I ran to greet them with my arms outstretched, crying delightedly, "You finally came!"

We went through ten pairs of missionaries in the next three years. My son and daughter and I were eager to be baptized, but Hal dragged his feet. He was converted, as were we, but somehow he couldn't make the commitment.

One morning as she was getting ready to go to school, our daughter, Wendy, who was about eleven years old and prone to being dramatic at times, made an announcement. "I've decided— I'm going to drink and smoke!" she said. And so saying, she flounced out the front door.

Hal sat quietly for a minute or two, then said, "Barbara, call the missionaries. We're going to be baptized."

As this chapter is being written, Wendy is serving a mission in Honduras; John has completed his mission in Argentina and has attended Brigham Young University. Would I have believed all this in my darkest days?

My dear friend Helen Wells, wife of Elder Robert E. Wells of the First Quorum of the Seventy, has written:

"Because of my husband's calling as a General Authority, some people say, 'What do you know about difficulties? You've got it made. You don't understand what we're going through.' Not many know how trying and difficult my journey has been at times. I know what it is like to be a single parent. I know what it is like to live thousands of miles away from parents, family, and friends. When I married Robert, I accepted three of his children, two of whom I'd never met.

"Anyone who becomes a parent to someone else's children knows the challenges that brings. Should I discipline them as I would my own? Should I treat them as though I were a visitor? Being human, I dealt with a 'ghost' — my husband's first wife, who in my mind undoubtedly was super-perfect.

"We spent a lot of time in South America. In Paraguay, I suffered through such intense heat that I had a miscarriage; and when I was carrying our daughter Sharlene [Miss America 1985], I threatened miscarriage two different times.

"In Cordoba, Argentina, I gave birth to Elayne; and one year later, while caring for little six-year-old Dana, whom we almost lost from appendicitis and peritonitis, I had another miscarriage.

"In Quito, Ecuador, the altitude was so high that during my pregnancy with Janet, Bob had to take me to Guayaquil on the coast so I could breathe. The problem became so pronounced that some months after the birth of Janet, the doctor ordered me to the States for an indefinite period. Our family was separated for three months, until one day Bob called to tell me he had been called to serve as mission president in Monterrey, Mexico.

"There have been other, even more difficult times over the years that have tested my soul to its very depth, though as I reflect back, the goodness of the Lord has softened those periods to the point that now I don't feel they were insurmountable.

"My only safe anchor from the storms of life is faith, and trust in God's will and mercy.

"A close friend wrote a beautiful message for her son and his friends. She shared that message with me, and I'll share excerpts from it with you:

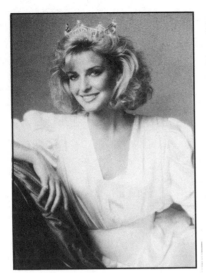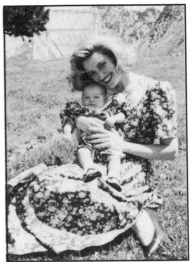

Sharlene Wells Hawkes: Miss America 1985 and loving mother
of Monica, born in March 1991

There is a reason to life. We can lift ourselves to heights we ourselves determine. We are filled with potential for excellence. We are free. We can learn to fly! Some cannot see — or may refuse to believe — the glory of the flight that awaits them. Spread wide your wings. Soar and try. Rise and guide yourself instead of going whither the wind blows.

> *The eagle knows that the higher he flies,*
> *The greater fulfillment, the brighter the skies.*
> *So look to your future with an eagle's eye.*
> *Believe in yourself—see how high you can fly.*

"To trust in God is to have faith in his plan for each of us, faith enough to have patience to endure disappointments and delays, confident that his perspective is much greater than ours. To achieve that level of confidence which allows us to be free of inner doubts and insecurities, we must have the faith and courage to believe in ourselves, realizing we come from royal lineage."

Never forget that we—you and I—are of royal lineage, and if we live worthily, one day in the eternities we may be queens.

Have you received the peace that comes from making contact with your Heavenly Father? Christ said, "Lo, I am with you alway, even unto the end of the world." (Matthew 28:20.) Pray and ask Him if you are doing His will. Ask in faith, nothing wavering. I can't promise you He will answer on a specific date. Like me, you may have to wait for His timetable. But I can guarantee that He does hear, that He will answer, and that His answer will be worth the wait.

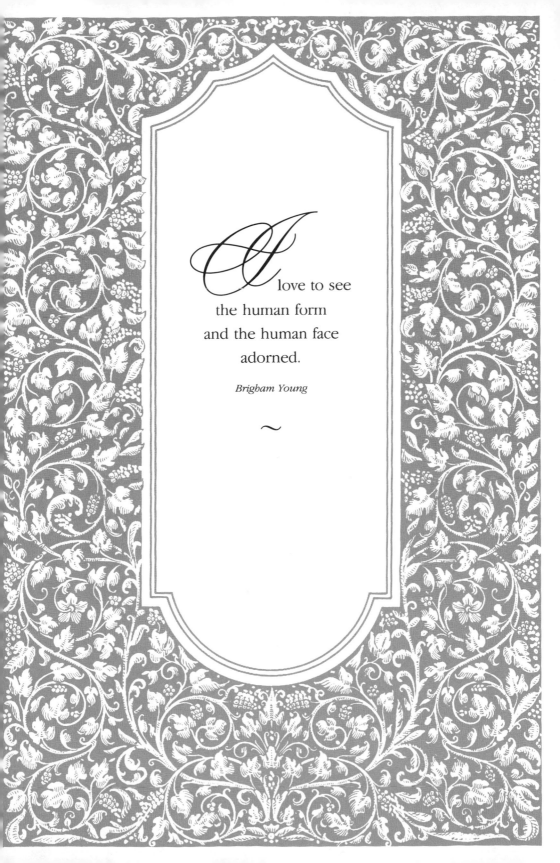

I love to see
the human form
and the human face
adorned.

Brigham Young

~

6

Fashion Changes — Style Remains

Brigham Young recognized that people feel good when they are dressed well, particularly when they do not follow the dictates of fashion, but select styles that are becoming to themselves. I like three statements he made: "Create your own fashions, and make your clothing to please yourselves, independent of outside influences." "In the works of God, you see an eternal variety, consequently we do not ask . . . the ladies [to] wear drab bonnets projecting in the front . . . with a cape behind." "Make your clothes suitable and becoming."

Coco Chanel, one of the greatest names in the fashion industry, once commented, "Fashion changes — style remains." Each of us is born with a distinctive personal style that is ours for life, despite the fickleness of changing hemlines or fashions that are here today and gone tomorrow. Whether we are aware of it or not, we each bear our own individual style, our own fashion personality.

Designers have identified six basic personal styles that describe one's personality, makeup, hair, and clothing. These styles are described on pages 58 to 63. See which one fits you best.

There are no preferred categories. Individual suitability is what counts. For instance, I am a Classic with a splash of Dramatic. (Women are usually dominant in one category, with undertones

(text continues on page 64)

57

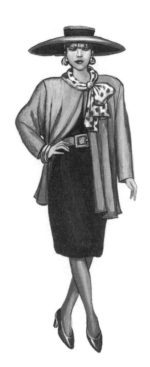
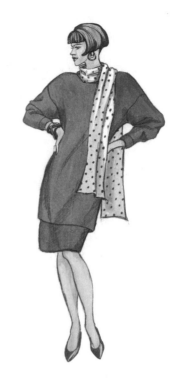

DRAMATIC

Words that describe you: Sophisticated, innovative, confident, bold, possibly even flamboyant.

Personality: Tendency to stand out, to be unique and original; capable; admired for style and often emulated.

Make-up: Usually dramatic; willing to try new techniques in private and use them in public only when they are perfected.

Hair: Interested in new styles, particularly sleek and away from the face.

Clothing: Concerned with style and trends, but not with fads; if style is right, it keeps long after it is no longer in fashion; bold colors; hats and turbans.

Pattern choices: Bold, such as dramatic florals, wide stripes, oversized dots, showy plaids.

Accessories: Unusual, such as one-of-a-kind pins; odd things used for different purposes, such as old belt buckle as a hair ornament.

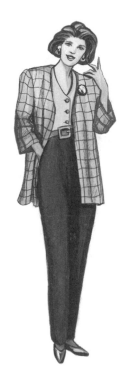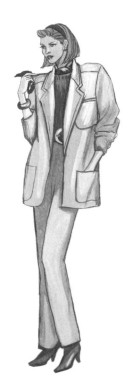

SPORTY

Words that describe you: Energetic, "All-American girl," easy to be
 with, high-spirited, dependable.

Personality: A spirited approach to life; natural and unpretentious;
 more comfortable at small, intimate parties than big gatherings.

Make-up: Natural-looking, leaning toward earth tones; because of
 life-style, may overdo for a formal occasion.

Hair: Always washed, clean; swingy and bouncy; easy-to-care-for style,
 perhaps blunt cut.

Clothing: Comfortable styles, to keep up with energetic life-style;
 tailored and conservative; wrinkle-resistant materials; tweeds,
 leather, suede, plaids; boots.

Pattern choices: Tartan plaids, muted stripes on wool, vague dots on
 tweedy fabrics, small floral designs

Accessories: Plain and few—small gold earrings, a nice pin, a leather
 belt, a necklace of wood.

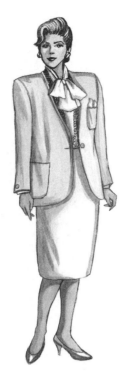 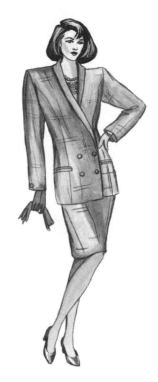

CLASSIC

Words that describe you: Elegant, calm, poised, classy, in control, organized, charming, perfectionist.

Personality: Admired and often emulated by others; able to accomplish much, which sometimes intimidates others; respected.

Make-up: Carefully crafted but never overdone or overstated; eye make-up complements outfit.

Hair: Never fussy or too curly: always clean, neatly shaped, medium length; style rarely changes.

Clothes: Rich-looking and elegant; feminine but tailored; fashions that never go out of style, such as suits and classic dresses.

Pattern choices: Solids rather than prints; occasional conservative geometric prints but usually no florals.

Accessories: Selected with care for each outfit — a single flower or beautiful pin; pearls; understated, classic, elegant.

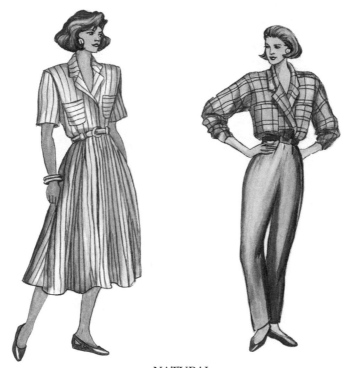

NATURAL

Words that describe you: Easy-going, casual, practical, natural, informal, unaffected.

Personality: Unpretentious and genuine; neat and uncluttered lifestyle; person to whom people are drawn; genuinely interested in others.

Make-up: Preference is to wear no make-up; for special occasions, a little foundation, blush, mascara, lipstick.

Hair: Casual, natural styles, either long or short; sometimes windblown styles or styles with curls close to head.

Clothing: Tailored, casual, comfortable; fabrics that require minimal care; youthful look; conservative; neutral colors.

Pattern choices: Solids or small-scale and detailed checks, plaids, dots, stripes, and florals.

Accessories: Kept to minimum, small, natural looking.

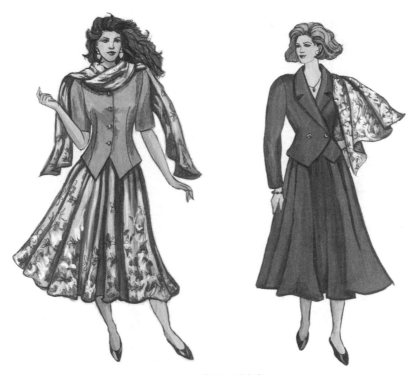

ROMANTIC

Words that describe you: Soft, loving, sentimental, tender, devoted,
   feminine, affectionate.

Personality: Charming, graceful, softly sophisticated; tendency toward
   hour-glass figure; "homey" life-style.

Make-up: Soft, smoky look in grays and pastels; no harsh lines; natural but softly radiant.

Hair: Softly curled, whether long or short.

Clothes: Pastels and soft fabrics; skirts rather than pants; pearls rather
   than gold; pale blue rather than electric blue; full rather than tailored skirts; never severe, starched, or crisp.

Pattern choices: Plain, soft solids; florals; softly blended geometrics and
   plaids; lacy; thin stripes.

Accessories: Medium-sized with dainty detail; small pearl earrings; de-
   mure gold locket.

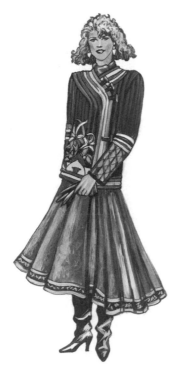 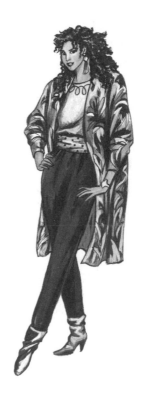

ARTY

Words that describe you: Free-spirited, individualistic, private, unique,
artistic, creative, thrifty, interesting.

Personality: A true individualist; private and unrushed; unique, personal mementos and furnishings preferred in home.

Make-up: Either none or lots, depending on occasion; focus on eyes;
dramatic look.

Hair: Individual look in any style, but possibly long and permed; natural color, perhaps with unusual highlights.

Clothes: Eye-catching and perhaps theatrical; natural fibers and tex-
ture; individualistic look, with unusual combinations; often purchased secondhand from thrift shops or flea markets.

Pattern choices: Mixed, from dramatic dots to romantic flowers, to create personal look.

Accessories: Quaint, uncommon pieces and combinations.

(text continued from page 57)

in another.) Kris Mackay is Romantic all the way. When we travel together to fulfill speaking engagements, we feel that we complement each other. But one thing we could never share (even if we were exactly the same size and so inclined) would be our clothes. Our styles are totally opposite. The soft, draped effect that is best for Kris would do nothing for me, and my crisp, tailored suits would appear too harsh on her.

Finding Your Personal Style

By now you probably suspect which fashion category fits you. To be certain, go through some fashion magazines and find illustrations of clothes that you especially like. (Don't skimp! This may be your one opportunity to put together your dream wardrobe with no restrictions as to cost.)

Cut out the illustrations and spread them out on a table. Scrutinize them carefully. Then reread the descriptions of the various fashion categories. Do you consistently lean toward crispness, or toward flowing lines? Is the jewelry that catches your eye large and dominant, or is it soft-spoken? Or do you prefer none at all? Remember to check out hairdos on the pictures you like. A definite motif will run through the assortment, and when you have finished, you should be fairly confident and ready to move to the next step—taking care of the things already in your wardrobe. Don't wait, promising yourself you'll tackle your wardrobe when you have lost those extra pounds. Begin today.

First, box up and get rid of everything you haven't worn for two years. Send these items to a thrift store, where they will be put to good use. I have known women in their twenties or even thirties who have hung onto a favorite skirt worn as a high school freshman. I've done it myself. If you must keep the skirt, wrap it in moth balls and store it away as a souvenir.

Next, box up items you have not worn for a year. These clothes may be perfectly smashing for someone else, but after ignoring them for a year, it is fairly certain that you do not feel quite right wearing them. You will probably never wear them again, but keep them stored away until you can face giving them away.

Then separate out those items that should be washed, mended, ironed, or sent to the cleaners, and shoes that could use a trip to the shoe repair shop (and please don't discard what is salvageable if it can be coupled with the right accessories). Take care of these problems immediately. Nothing is more frustrating than to reach for a favorite pair of slacks and find a split seam or a spot on one leg.

After discarding things you no longer wear, and freshening and repairing each remaining garment, proceed to organize your closet according to skirts, blouses, dresses, and so on.

Now make note of all the different combinations you can use: the black skirt with the green blouse and paisley scarf; the black skirt with the white blouse and big silver belt. You get the idea. How many times have you opened your closet door and moaned, "I have absolutely nothing to wear"? With a little creative planning, you will be amazed at how many outfits you can put together before you buy something new.

Stop and think before you buy. You are a wise shopper only if you have learned that fashion is a way of looking, not a price. On a budget, the trick is to select new clothes that look expensive but aren't.

Go to a department or specialty women's store and analyze the look of expensive clothes sold there—the cut, the fabric, the workmanship, and the details. Try some on. There's no law against looking. Once you develop an eye for real quality, you will recognize its look in lower-priced garments.

Unless you have absolutely unlimited funds, the way to create a wardrobe with the right clothes for every occasion is to plan ahead. Make no spur-of-the-moment purchases that ruin your budget and merely take up space in your closet; unconsidered selections often aren't your style, and you probably won't enjoy wearing them.

In chapter 3, we discussed color. By now you know whether you are "warm" or "cool," and nowhere is that information more important to follow than in selecting new clothes. Coordinating color to your skin tone is one of the most crucial beauty aids available. If it will help you, purchase a paperback book on color and take it with you when shopping, to keep you on the right track.

Your best purchase is something I refer to as a best basic, that is, a simple basic dress or suit with versatile, unadorned lines in one of your colors. Using scarves, belts, jewelry, and other accessories, this classic basic can be adapted to fit every fashion personality.

Scarves can dress up and add a flair to even the plainest clothes. And you can make them with one yard of polyester silk (which is generally inexpensive and washable) from a fabric store. One day in a store in San Francisco, I saw a beautiful silk scarf with tassels that I fell in love with, but the price was an astronomical $160. So I bought a yard of polyester silk for $6.98 and three tassels for $1.98 each. I folded the silk into an inside-out triangle, sewed the edges, turned it right-side out, and added the three tassels, one at each point. For an elegant finishing touch, hem your scarf by hand. The total cost of my new scarf was less than one-tenth the cost of the scarf in the store.

Illustrations on pages 67 to 69 show several ways to tie your scarf, using scarf clips. A scarf can also make a beautiful alternative to wearing a necklace. Fold the scarf into its longest length, knot it in the center, and tie the two ends at the back of your neck.

Other accessories can also be made inexpensively at home to give your outfit individual flair. Once I needed some earrings to match an outfit I already had. I bought a pair on sale for $2.00, even though they were the wrong color. I painted them myself, using an old eyeshadow brush, with airplane paint (available in a drugstore). They looked beautiful — and expensive. You can also cover undecorated earrings (look for them in a fabric store) with material from the ends of the scarf fabric you purchased, for almost instant coordination.

I believe that women make more mistakes with shoes than with any other piece of clothing. The effect of a beautifully as-

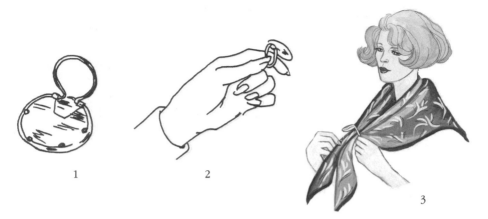

The Scarf Shawl: (1) Open ring at back of clip. (2) Hold ring, using thumb and index finger, and (3) slip scarf through ring. Snap ring to fasten.

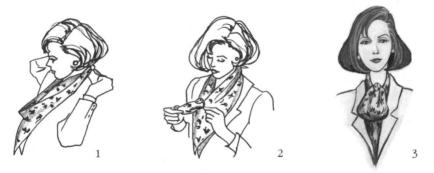

The Suit Filler: (1) Fold a square scarf into a triangle. Place points in front and tie ends at back of neck. (2) Pull about 5 inches of the center of the scarf through the center of the scarf clip. Fasten clip. Slide clip up to neck by gently pulling fabric to form a pouf. (3) Tuck remaining fabric to fill in neckline.

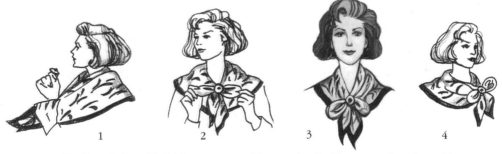

The Bow Collar: (1) Fold a square scarf into a triangle. Place over shoulders with triangle points in back. Pull middle (not ends) of fabric through ring of clip. (2) Fasten clip and adjust loops on either side to form a bow. (3) Wear bow in front or (4) to the side.

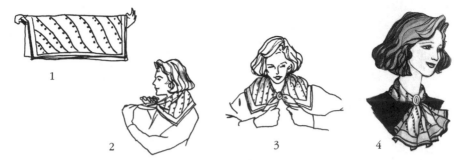

The Jabot: (1) Fold a square scarf in half to form a rectangle. (2) Place scarf over shoulders with ends meeting. Place ends through ring and slide clip up to neck. (3) Fasten clip. Pull ends of scarf, from inside edges, to fan out. (4) Wear clip in front to form a jabot, or wear it to the side.

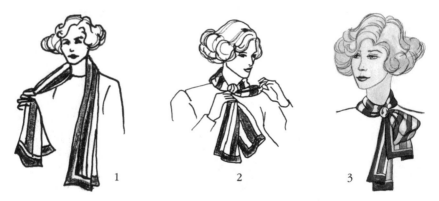

The Assymetric Bow: (1) Place oblong scarf around neck. Pull one end of the scarf through ring approximately two-thirds of the way up. (2) Pinch center of opposite side, level with the clip. Pull loop through ring. (3) Fasten clip and adjust.

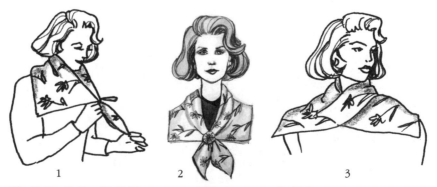

The Sailor Collar: (1) Fold a square scarf into a rectangle. Pick up two opposite corners to form two triangles. Place scarf around neck and pull ends through scarf ring. Slide clip up and fasten. (2) Spread each panel to create a "sailor collar." (3) As a variation, turn clip around to back for a soft drape look in front.

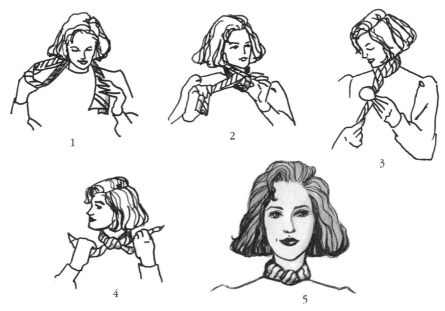

The Choker: (1) Fold an oblong scarf in half. Place around neck, holding loop in one hand and ends in other. (2) Pull ends through loop and tighten at neck. (3) Slide scarf clip on ends and push up to loop. (4) Tuck ends of scarf in toward back of neck. (5) Wear scarf with bare neck or with blouse or dress.

sembled outfit can be ruined if you wear the wrong pair of shoes with it. Just because feet are down on the ground below eye level doesn't mean people don't notice them.

Don't always try to match your shoes to the color of your clothing, but do harmonize. Wear shoes that are a color value that is the same as or darker than the color at your hemline (exception: never wear black or brown shoes with a white or solid beige outfit). Keeping your shoes the same color or darker gives a nice flow to your outfit and balance to your body, keeps you grounded, and does not draw the eye too quickly to your feet (usually not one's best asset). However, fabric pumps dyed to match the fabric of a dress are recommended only for very dressy evening occasions or weddings.

Be careful about wearing white shoes. An old rule, one that I still consider to be valid, is this: White shoes should be worn only from May to Labor Day except in a warm climate, such as

Hawaii. For the remainder of the year, if you wear a winter-white ensemble, you should wear winter-white (off-white) shoes to match.

Also, be cautious about wearing white or ivory-colored hosiery. Lightness increases the perception of heavy calves.

By now you may feel like setting a match to your current wardrobe. Don't! Work with what you have. If a garment is the wrong color, make it work for you by adding scarves or accessories in your right colors. The important thing is that the colors that are most flattering to you be nearest your face.

Several times I have alluded to the word *flair*. Flair is that little extra something that makes a woman look memorable. The dictionary defines flair as "an instinctive ability to appreciate or make good use of something; talent; a uniquely attractive quality." Flair gives you a well-dressed look indelibly stamped with your name. And it can be acquired through conscious effort. Although some people have flair instinctively — and to a certain extent most women do lean toward whichever of the fashion categories suits their personal style best — I cannot stress enough how important it is for the confident woman to identify her own personal style and make the most of it.

So get out those scissors, and start putting together your dream wardrobe!

7

The Face of a Queen

Though Brigham Young lived more than a century ago, he certainly understood many things that medical science and beauty experts have taught in recent years, as these statements illustrate: "Study to preserve the skin from being ruined by dirt, and the heat of the scorching sun" and "Make your hats and bonnets to shade you." He also said, "I love to see . . . the human face adorned."

Beauty doesn't necessarily equate with spending money. There are many things any woman can do to take care of and pamper herself, using items found in every kitchen.

My favorite skin-care treat is called "Princess Grace's Secret Rosewater." Fill a pot with wilted rose petals. Pour purified water to the top of the pan. Simmer on low heat until the petals are "mushy," approximately 20 to 30 minutes. (If you prefer, microwave the petals for approximately 10 minutes.) Strain the liquid and put it in a clean spray bottle. Spray your face or body before applying facial moisturizer or body creams. You will notice a dramatic difference in the softness of your skin.

Daily Skin Care

1. Each morning, cleanse your skin to help prevent complications from heavy buildup of makeup, excess oils, and impurities from the air, and to remove waste and bacteria. I recommend using a cleansing gel. Soap removes bacteria in most cases, but

71

it isn't as effective in removing makeup and dead cells, and it often leaves a residue in the pores.

2. Use a toner (if you have normal skin) or an astringent (if your skin is oily) to prepare your skin for the moisturizer. Do not use alcohol.

3. Moisturize your skin to protect it from wind, dirt, and pollution. For normal skin, use a product that says "moisturizer" on the label. For oily skin, use "oil-free moisturizer." (Check to be sure your nourishing creams contain no fillers of petroleum or beeswax, since they block absorption.)

4. Apply makeup. (See figures 1 to 21.)

5. Every evening, repeat the process: cleanse, tone, and moisturize your skin as detailed above. Then, if your skin is dry, apply night cream to your entire face; if not, apply night cream only underneath eyes. Remember, the eye area has no natural oil glands.

Weekly Skin Care

1. Cleanse your skin, as described above.

2. Rinse your skin and then steam it to open the pores, make deep cleansing possible, and cleanse and relax the complexion.

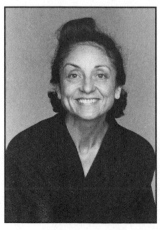 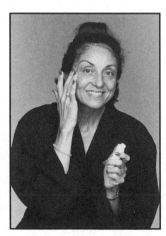 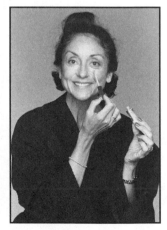

Making up your face: (1) Start with a clean face and spray with a fine mist of rosewater. (2) Apply thin coat of moisturizer (with sun factor of 15) over entire face. (3) Apply concealer (see figure 4) that is one-half shade lighter than foundation.

To give yourself a steam facial, fill a pot with water and bring it to a boil. (If you wish, you may add 1 tablespoon herbal tea leaves.) Remove the pan from the heat. Lean over the pot and drape a towel over your head and the pot, forming a tent. Steam your face for approximately five minutes, then rinse with cool water.

3. Exfoliate your skin to remove dead skin cells. I like to use a concoction that you can make at home, using sage (a natural astringent) and bran (which helps exfoliate dead or dry surface skin). In the top of a double boiler, melt 2 bars of high-quality glycerin soap, 1 ounce chopped fresh sage, 8 drops olive oil, and 1 tablespoon bran. Pour the mixture into waxed cupcake papers nestled in a cupcake pan. Let harden. Use to wash and exfoliate your face.

4. Use a mask to moisturize skin and tighten pores. Mix 2 teaspoons honey with 1 egg yolk. Smooth onto your face. Leave on approximately 20 minutes. Rinse with warm water.

5. Lubricate your face. Apply a thin layer (2 to 3 tablespoons)

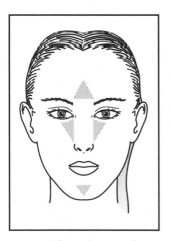 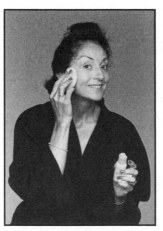 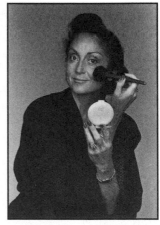

(4) Apply concealer to areas in triangles. Cover only darkest areas of under-eye circles, extending in an elongated triangle to tip of nose. (5) Apply sheer foundation that matches exactly color of skin tone at jaw line. Blend, especially into hair line. (6) Using fluffy brush, apply thin coat of translucent powder to entire face.

of slightly warm olive or cod-liver oil to dry areas of your face. Leave on for several hours. (For oily skin, use your oil-free moisturizer.)

Applying Makeup

Figures 1 to 21 illustrate steps to follow in making up your face. In these instructions, perhaps the most important word is *blend* — always using a sponge. There should never be any harsh lines in a makeup application.

As you are learning to apply makeup, you might want to go to three different cosmetic counters in a large department store (on three different days) and have a makeup expert at each make up your face. You may not like the results, but I promise you that you will learn something from each application that will help you to develop a better look and to become a more confident you.

One additional makeup tip: Recycle your old lipsticks. Purchase a small plastic bobbin box (available at fabric stores), and

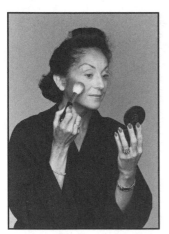 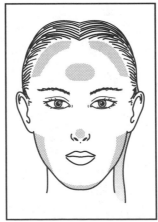 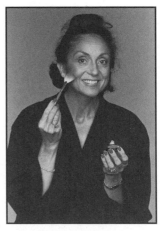

(7) If desired, to give your face a healthy glow and make it appear more oval in shape, brush bronzing powder *very sparingly* on cheeks, forehead, chin, and top of nose. (8) Shaded areas show where to apply bronzing powder. (9) Using a brush, apply blush along cheekbone, from center of ear toward tip of nose, stopping at imaginary line down from outside of pupil (see figure 10). Keep blush deeper and darker near ear. Blend. As you age, you may want to put small dot of blush under arch of brow to create softening effect.

put an old tube of lipstick in each slot. Then, using a lipbrush, you can combine the shades and make your own "new colors."

Caring for Your Hair

"Keep your hair smooth and nice. The hair is given to the female for adornment [meaning to add beauty]; and therefore let the ladies, young and old, adorn their heads with their hair," said Brigham Young.

No woman is ever completely satisfied with her own hair. It's always the wrong color, too straight or too curly, too dry or too oily, too thin or too thick. But there is hope for any type of hair if it is kept healthy, gleaming, and fashionably cut. Here are some tips for caring for your hair.

1. *Shampooing:* Start by changing your shampoo, and change it often. For best results, purchase your shampoos at a beauty-supply store or salon where the correct shampoos—those that are designed for your hair type and are pH-balanced—are sold.

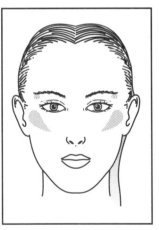 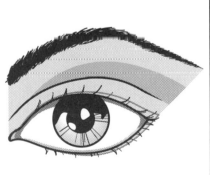 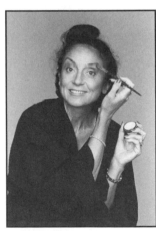

(10) Illustration shows placement of blush at cheekbones and under arch of brow. (11) Illustration shows placement of eye makeup (see figures 12–14). (12) Apply eyeshadow base over entire lid in a shade to complement skin tone.

I recommend that you don't use shampoos that are generally found at grocery stores, drugstores, or discount stores; those products can strip your hair of important natural oils.

2. *Moisturizing:* Use a small amount of moisturizer on the ends of your hair each time you shampoo. Most people need a good moisturizer rather than conditioner for general daily use, to protect their hair from the elements of nature.

3. *Conditioning:* Choose a conditioner that corresponds to your hair type and use it sparingly. A very small dab, about the size of a dime, is usually sufficient. Apply only to the ends; then rinse it out. Some people cannot use a conditioner because it makes their hair droopy. What's best for you? Ask a professional stylist.

4. *Final rinse:* Combine 1/2 cup white vinegar and 1/2 cup distilled water, and use as a hair toner after shampooing.

Treat your hair occasionally to a deep-conditioning treatment.

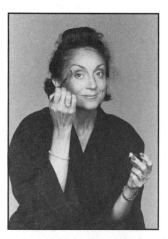 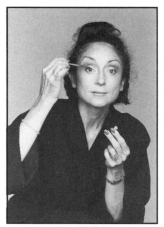 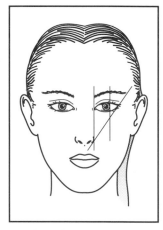

(13) Apply eyeshadow shading just above crease of eye, using a shade that blends with hair color but is not as dark as brows. (14) With a pencil, apply eye liner. Make small dots as close to lash line as possible; blend with cotton swab. With small wedge-shaped brush, line directly over pencil with powdered shadow that matches color of outer rim of iris; blend again. (15) Illustration shows placement of eyebrow makeup. Following diagram, measure brows for stragglers and to emphasize natural arch.

Here are some treatments that you can prepare easily at home. (Don't try them all in one day, as one woman did!)

1. To seal in natural moisture, shampoo your hair with a mixture of one-half ripe, mashed avocado combined with enough shampoo and water for one application. Then rinse well.

2. Combine 1 egg, 1 teaspoon honey, and 1 teaspoon olive oil. Massage into hair and scalp. Leave on for 20 minutes; then shampoo out.

3. Apply pure vegetable oil generously to hair; then wrap head in a hot towel (fresh from the dryer) or plastic wrap, to seal in body heat. Leave on hair for 30 minutes. Shampoo out.

4. Combine 2 ounces (about 4 tablespoons) mayonnaise with 1 tablespoon cider vinegar, and apply generously to hair. Massage gently into scalp. Wrap in plastic wrap to seal in body heat. Leave on hair for 30 minutes, then shampoo out.

Changing Your Hairstyle

How long has it been since you changed your hairstyle? Maybe it's time to make a change. So how do you go about doing this?

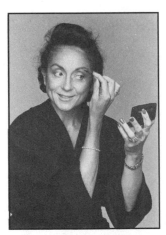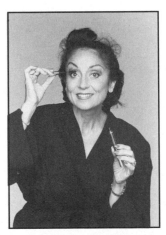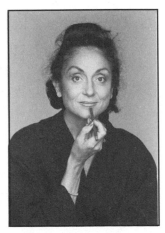

(16) Apply eyebrow makeup with small wedge-shaped brush in tiny hairlike stokes. If brows are thin, use cake-type eyebrow shadow to thicken. Finish with clear mascara to hold hairs in place (17) Apply mascara one shade darker than hair, to make lashes appear fuller. Be sure lashes don't clump together. (18) Outline lips with a lip pencil.

1. Collect pictures of hairstyles you like as well as those you don't like. Select two or three that you especially like.

2. Find a good hairstylist. If you see someone whose hairstyle you like, ask her who her stylist is. She will be complimented that you asked. If you live in a city, call the society editor of your local newspaper. Explain your dilemma and ask for a recommendation. You will be surprised at how helpful she will be, at least if your experience is anything like mine.

4. Before making an appointment to have your hair done, interview the stylist or stylists on your list. Most stylists will agree to do a consultation free of charge. Explain to them your lifestyle, show them the two or three pictures of hairstyles you like, and ask them what they would do with your hair. If your hair is graying or you are unhappy with your color, ask for suggestions on how to handle such problems. If you like what you hear, schedule an appointment.

5. When you go to your appointment, be on time. You don't want the stylist to have to rush. Don't be afraid to ask questions regarding the care and maintenance of your new look. This can make all the difference in loving or hating your new style. Most important of all, give yourself enough time to get used to

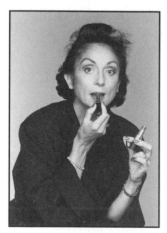 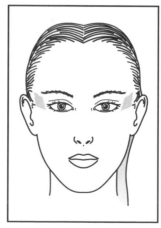 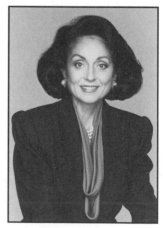

(19) Apply lipstick color within outline. Blend with foam tip end of an eyeliner pencil so that lip liner is not noticeable. (20) Apply concealer on temples, between eyes and hairline to create a more youthful illusion in the eye area. (21) Makeup is now complete.

the change. After a full week of compliments, you will wish you had changed your style sooner.

Pampering Your Body

Here are three ways to make your skin as soft as a baby's:

1. Combine 1 cup Epsom salt with liquid soap and a little water to make a thick paste. Using a loofah mitt or washcloth, apply paste over your entire body, rubbing vigorously to remove dead skin cells. Shower. Apply moisturizing cream to your skin.

2. Combine 1 egg yolk, 8 tablespoons baby oil, and 1 table-spoon cider vinegar. Apply mixture to entire body; leave on skin for 20 to 30 minutes. Rinse off in a quick, brisk shower. Then soak in a soothing milk bath.

3. For a milk bath, fill your bathtub with warm water, 85 to 95 degrees F. Add 1/2 cup milk and 2 capfuls oil (such as baby oil or coconut oil). Soak for 20 minutes. (Do not soak longer than 20 minutes or you may become dehydrated.)

Caring for Your Nails

If I were to neglect to mention the care of your fingernails, it would be like giving approval to serve a cake without icing at a birthday party. It is as important to have your nails in good condition as to have all the rest of you in elegant, queenly order.

You don't have to have long, crimson nails to look queenly; all you need is to keep your nails neatly filed in an oval shape, (use an emery board rather than a metal file) and to keep the cuticles pushed back with a cuticle stick and a little cuticle re-mover (which can be purchased at any drugstore).

To add the finishing touch, use some pretty polish in your choice of color. Polishes that contain nail tougheners are excellent for nails that are thin and weak.

I do not recommend acrylic nails because the chemicals can damage your natural nails, but if you would like to try something that will help you to have longer nails, here are two options:

1. Have your nails professionally wrapped with silk at a salon.

Your nails will not break, and the polish will last approximately four weeks.

2. For a do-it-yourself-at-home treatment, combine in a small glass jar 4 tablespoons white iodine (purchased at a pharmacy) and 4 tablespoons olive oil. Every night, wash your hands and apply a coat of clear polish to your nails. Then shake the iodine and oil mixture, and carefully dip each nail into it. (Yes, it works even with polish on your nails.) The iodine will toughen the nail fiber, and the olive oil will both soften your cuticles and act as an instant dryer for the polish. You can apply approximately fourteen layers of polish to your nails before removing the polish.

Always wear gloves when your hands are in water and when you garden. I promise you that if you take proper care of your nails, you will feel elegant, pampered, and special.

8

A Collage of Beauty Tips

Each of the young women I have worked with in preparing for pageants has special things she does to maintain her health and beauty. Five of these women have agreed to share with you some of their tips. Here they are, along with a word or two about what each one is doing with her life now that the pageant is over.

Laura Martinez-Herring, Miss USA 1985: "At 5:30 each morning, I get up and drive to the base of a nearby mountain, where I hike to the top. It takes me forty-five minutes uphill and twenty-five minutes down. That gets my circulation going, puts clean oxygen into my system, and gives my skin a radiant, healthy glow. It also allows me time to center on God. I feel incredible for the rest of the day.

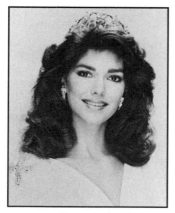

Laura Martinez-Herring
Miss USA 1985

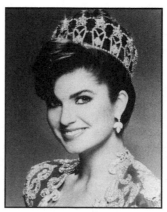

Michelle Royer Jefferson
Miss USA 1987

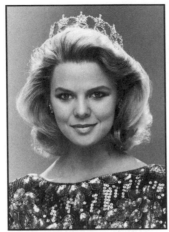

Christy Fichtner Alhadef
Miss USA 1986

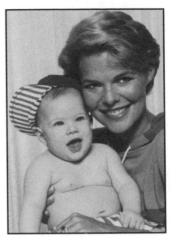

Christy Fichtner Alhadef
with baby son

"A cosmetic beauty tip? After cleansing my face, I drench a cotton ball with water, squeeze it out, add a little rice vinegar, and smooth it all over my face. Then I apply a moisturizer. I use all-natural beauty products, but I recommend this rice-vinegar toner especially."

Laura is presently making her way into movies and TV and recently played a role on "General Hospital." She is continuing to learn about the importance of attitude, believing that we each can choose how we will react to anything. She has learned to accept loss as an indication that it's time to move on to a new chapter in her life. She feels that the most important thing is to center on and stay close to God.

Christy Fichtner Alhadef, Miss USA 1986: "It's important to organize your life so you can find time to take care of yourself. I am married to a dentist and am the mother of a young son. When Barbara called, I was rushing out the door to a modeling job. Being a mother, which I love, I find I must be organized. The first thing I do early each morning is make myself look good. If I don't put on makeup and do my hair, I feel dowdy, and my day is never as productive."

Christy practices what she preaches. Although her son is still

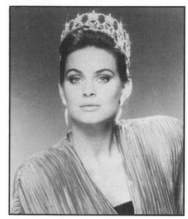

Courtney Gibbs
Miss USA 1988

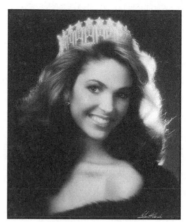

Gretchen Polhemus
Miss USA 1989

very young, she is already back to a size 5. She makes certain that when opportunities come her way, she is ready.

Michelle Royer Jefferson, Miss USA 1987: "My most important tip is to throw away the scales. Eat only when you are hungry, not just because it's time to eat or because everyone else is eating. Don't deprive yourself of something you crave. Eat just a small amount, but don't go overboard.

"I have very sensitive skin, so I use baby soap, baby lotion, and Lubriderm as a moisturizer. When I'm headed for an exercise class and don't want to put on full makeup, I use a little concealer on dark eye circles or shadows and a little blush on eyelids and cheeks. I finish with a bit of mascara and lip gloss."

Michelle, who also does aerobics three days a week, is currently working on a degree in journalism and hosts a TV talk show. She is married to a radio disc jockey.

Courtney Gibbs, Miss USA 1988: "I always wear sun screen, even if I don't plan to go outside. Even the ultraviolet rays of indoor lighting damage the skin. Many makeup lines offer a facial moisturizer that contains a sun block. A number 15 is recommended.

"Another secret is to get outside sometime every day and take a brisk walk, ride a bike, or play tennis. It's important to be out in the fresh air, to smell the grass and flowers, to hear the birds singing, and to look at the trees. It makes me feel better all day."

Courtney is one of the top models in Los Angeles and a national spokesperson for a major diet-drink firm. She recently moved to the beach, where she can enjoy lots of fresh air and commune with nature.

Gretchen Polhemus, Miss USA 1989: "We can't undo damage already done to our skin, but we can help prevent what's about to happen. I've started to take extra care of my skin by using under-eye, throat, and lip creams at night, and lotion on my hands. I recommend a gel cleanser and a toner. About once a week I massage cornmeal, moistened with gel, on my face to get rid of dead skin cells."

Gretchen is currently a spokeswoman for an ESPN television program.

Tips from the Pros

I've worked for years with Guyrex Associates, a firm that has coached six Miss USA winners and countless other beauty pageant contestants on how to walk into a room and light it up with a dazzling smile, a terrific appearance, and, even more important, supreme self-confidence. An article in *Woman's Day* (September 4, 1990) tells how a busy radiologist, Gabriela Kaplan, flew to El Paso to spend a day with Guyrex image consultants—not to become a contestant but because she wished to present herself more effectively to patients and at occasional speaking engagements. In the magazine she listed what helped her the most: "I wear shoulder pads and watch my posture to make myself seem taller. I turn my collars up, push my sleeves up, do everything I can to get an *up* line, because Guyrex made me see how things sag as we get older." She listed some of Guyrex's tips, including the following:

1. "Keep skin hydrated. Drink water, steam your face, invest in a humidifier." (Moisturize with the rosewater I told you how to prepare in chapter 7.)

2. "If your hair suffers from mishandling, wear it pulled up

until it restores itself." (I like to point out that God made our bodies with the miraculous quality of self-healing. If we take care of ourselves, nature will do its part.)

3. "For quick energy and a rosy glow, bend over from the waist and hold your breath for 15 seconds."

4. "Make a habit of tightening tummy muscles whenever the thought occurs to you."

5. "Keep in mind that of all the things you wear, your expression counts the most."

Dr. Kaplan had no problem grasping that last suggestion. Her final comment was: "But the most important thing I learned, and I know this sounds corny, is attitude. *People will see you as pretty if you make them feel good.*"

My Daily Routine

As I speak with women all over the country, many ask what I personally do each day. Here is my typical routine.

After rising, I cleanse and moisturize my skin, eat three prunes, drink 4 ounces of unfiltered apple juice, and take vitamins.

I do thirty minutes of stomach-tightening and slow, limbering stretches while watching the news on television.

For breakfast I have two-thirds cup of bran cereal with fresh fruit and a cup of cinnamon-apple herb tea.

My lunch is a sandwich of either turkey or vegetables on whole-grain bread. My beverage is always calorie-free.

At four o'clock I snack on a plain bagel with no butter or cream cheese.

In the late afternoon or early evening, I walk on my treadmill for forty-five minutes, six days a week, while watching an educational video or listening to an educational tape. Upbeat music in the background makes walking easier.

For dinner, I have a huge serving of my power salad (recipe in chapter 12), 4 ounces of fresh fish, a generous serving of steamed vegetables, mineral water with lemon, and a low-calorie dessert. (Sometimes I eat two *real* cookies. I'm not perfect!) I have a passion for Mexican food and pizza, but when I indulge, it is the exception to the rule and not the rule.

At this stage of my life, I don't follow this daily routine to further a career in ballet. Now my main priority is a personal need to remain limber and to just plain feel good and have an abundance of energy. Do you feel the same needs? Stretching, exercising, and healthful eating will help!

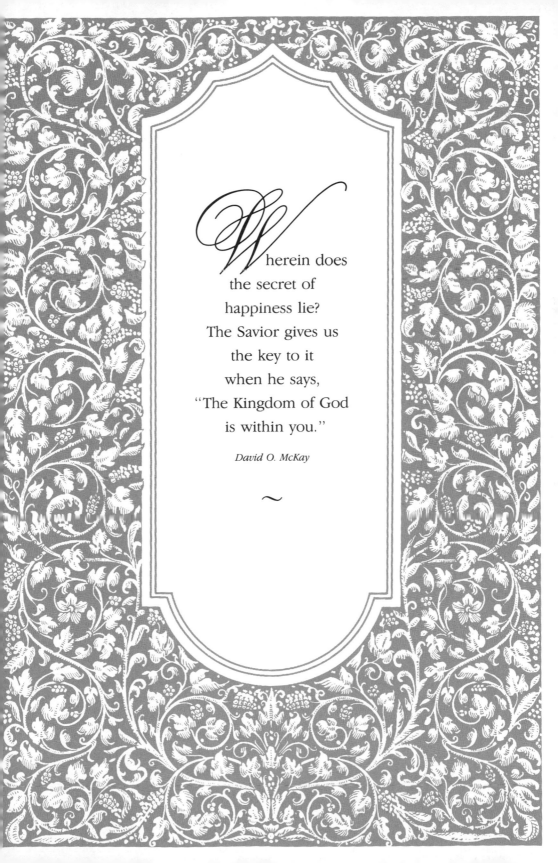

Wherein does
the secret of
happiness lie?
The Savior gives us
the key to it
when he says,
"The Kingdom of God
is within you."

David O. McKay

~

9

Make the Best of Your Circumstances

Recently I received a letter from a teenager in which she poured out her feelings in seven pages of searing self-hatred. Here are some of the things she told me:

"I hate everything about myself, physically, mentally, spiritually, and socially. I study everyone around me and they are so superior that jealousy makes me feel depressed and hopeless. My hands are short and stubby, my fingers fat and kind of crooked. The rest of my body is grotesque.

"I play the piano, but no better than average. I love to sing, but there are voices better than mine. I went to my little sister's dance recital and ended up hating my mother because she didn't bother to let me study ballet.

"Life is an unorganized disaster. Every goal I set I end up breaking, so I rip myself apart further for not following through. I know about positive attitude, but gosh, Sister Jones, this is supposed to be the dispensation for incredibly special spirits. What am I doing here on earth?"

After signing her name, she added a postscript: "Please write me back. I need to know that if I try again, you think this time it can be different."

When I read her letter, I felt like crying. That letter is a classic example of the danger of comparing yourself with someone else and finding yourself unnaturally wanting.

Have you ever said to yourself, when things weren't going

quite as you wished they would, words to this effect: "Oh, if only..." or "Someday..." or "When this or that happens, then...."? An unknown poet once described this tendency so many people have of not being satisfied with what is happening in the present, of always looking for something else to happen so they can be happy:

> *It was spring, but it was summer I wanted—*
> *The warm days, the great outdoors.*
> *It was summer, but it was fall I wanted—*
> *The colorful leaves, the cold, dry air.*
> *It was fall, but it was winter I wanted—*
> *The beautiful snow, the joy of the holiday season.*
> *It was winter, but it was spring I wanted—*
> *The warmth, the blossoming of nature.*
>
> *I was a child, but it was adulthood I wanted—*
> *The freedom, the respect.*
> *I was twenty, but it was thirty I wanted—*
> *To be mature and sophisticated.*
> *I was middle-aged, but it was twenty I wanted—*
> *The youth, the free spirit.*
> *I was retired, but it was middle-age I wanted—*
> *The presence of mind without limitations.*
>
> *My life was over.*
> *I never got what I wanted.*

Some time ago a woman who signed herself "Heartsick" wrote the following letter to advice columnist Ann Landers:

"My handsome, successful, workaholic husband just learned he has cancer. His chances for making it are about 50–50. I am trying to be brave for him, and he is putting on the same act for me. A while back you ran an essay called 'The Station.' It was about how we all have a tendency to put things off, not enjoying the journey through life because we focus on the destination that is always somewhere ahead. Please rerun that essay, Ann. It may help someone else."

Ann Landers reprinted the essay, which was written by Robert J. Hastings.[1] Mr. Hastings might have written his essay with me in mind. Here is how it begins:

"Tucked away in our subconscious is an idyllic vision. We see ourselves on a long trip that spans the continent. We are traveling by train. Out the windows we drink in the passing scene of cars on nearby highways, of children waving at a crossing, of cattle grazing on a distant hillside. . . .

"But uppermost in our minds is the final destination. On a certain day at a certain hour we will pull into the station. Bands will be playing and flags waving. Once we get there so many wonderful dreams will come true and the pieces of our lives will fit together like a completed jigsaw puzzle. We pace the aisles, waiting, waiting, waiting for the station.

" 'When we reach the station, that will be it!' we cry. . . . "

When I was a gawky child, I thought, "When I am in high school, I will be beautiful and popular. Life will be different." I reached my teenage years and thought, "This isn't what I expected. When I go to New York to study ballet, then I will be happy."

In New York I saw all the beautiful ballerinas, so thin, so glamorous. I was scared and homesick. At first I was so overwhelmed that I turned to eating to console myself. I gained weight, and the school threatened to send me home. I thought, "When I am thin again, everything will be okay." I went on a starvation diet and started gulping down laxatives. I grew skeleton thin, but had to go home anyway because I became anemic. I had no doubt that my life was over.

Back home, all my friends were married. I told myself, "When I'm married, then I will be happy." I accepted a ring from a young man I had known and loved for years. We sent out wedding invitations, my dress was hanging in the closet, and the gifts sparkled on our dining room table. One week before the wedding, I could tell something was wrong. My fiancé didn't look me in the eye; he didn't kiss me goodnight. It wasn't working. We called the wedding off.

I was devastated. Then his best friend asked me to marry him. My heart was set on being married, so I agreed. As somebody's wife, surely I would reach the "station" where the band would play and the flags would wave. You already know how that turned out. (See chapter 5.)

Married and miserable, I longed to be free. I ran away, even from my baby, but my "station" wasn't there either. If only I had my baby back, I thought, that would be enough. That would be all I needed.

I got him back. We lived in Canada in tenement housing, and I didn't have enough money to buy my baby's milk. I told myself, "When I can give my son a backyard to play in, and a dog . . ." So I went back to my husband, to a house with a yard and a dog, but the contentment I had spent my life waiting for still eluded me.

"The Station" continues:

"Sooner or later we must realize there is no station, no one place to arrive at once and for all. The true joy of life is the trip. The station is only a dream. It constantly outdistances us.

" 'Relish the moment' is a good motto, especially when coupled with Psalm 118:24: 'This is the day which the Lord hath made; we will rejoice and be glad in it.' It isn't the burdens of today that drive men mad. It is the regrets over yesterday and the fear of tomorrow. Regret and fear are twin thieves who rob us of today."

To remind us to count our blessings, I have developed a chart that I call "Happiness/Misery Index." The top half of the chart reminds us to keep our focus on God and His Son, Jesus Christ. To do that, we must live in a positive way, which in turn will nurture a positive ego; indulging in self-pity and negative thoughts and actions will only lead to negative ego. In other words, we must have hope, not worry; enthusiasm, not discouragement; faith, not doubt; and love, not despair. Love, faith, enthusiasm, and hope lead to God and Christ; the baser emotions — worry, discouragement, doubt, and despair — are tools of Satan.

1. We can remain the same and wallow in the comfort of discomfort (misery) — or we can work to change ourselves (happiness).

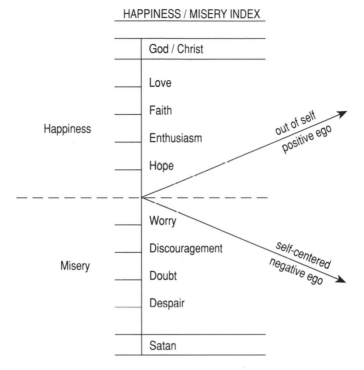

HAPPINESS / MISERY INDEX

2. We can be grouchy (misery) — or we can look at the lighter side of life and have a sense of humor (happiness).

3. We can say, "My will be done" (misery) — or we can say, and act, to back up our words, "Thy will be done" (happiness).

4. We can say "If only . . ." (misery) — or we can make the best of our circumstances (happiness).

5. We can submit to stress and burnout (misery) — or we can take care of ourselves and enjoy inner peace (happiness).

6. We can sit around and feel sluggish (misery) — or we can exercise and feel more energetic (happiness).

7. We can eat the wrong kinds of foods and feel sluggish and gain weight (misery) — or we can eat the proper foods and feel more energetic and lose weight (happiness).

8. We can succumb to addictions (misery) — or we can develop self-discipline (happiness).

9. We can look for instant gratification (misery) — or we can

be willing to do whatever is necessary and right in order to achieve what we really want to achieve (happiness).

When Hal and I were married, he said to me, "Look, I am 80 percent good and 20 percent not-so-good. If you choose to focus on my 80 percent, we will get along fine. If you focus on my not-so-good 20 percent, we may end up getting a divorce." I was startled, to say the least. Then he explained, "That's the way it is with most things — 80 percent good and 20 percent not-so-good. How we conduct our lives, our happiness or lack thereof, depends on our attitude. We all have to make the choice."

As we strive to be women of confidence, to be queens, we must also choose to exhibit kindness toward ourselves. The critical, heartless way some women view themselves has very little to do with who they really are. For example, women who suffer from anorexia look in the mirror and see fat that simply is not there.

Wouldn't it be wonderful if we could all look at our circumstances with the faith and enthusiasm of Jean VanTrump, whom I met at a meeting at which I spoke. Jean is a woman with real problems, but she still looks at the 80 percent that is good. This note from her was like a breath of fresh air:

"I am the one in the Palm Beach Gardens chapel who was in the wheelchair. As I spoke to you then, I asked that you help others who are in a similar situation to mine, help them to feel as good about themselves as I feel about myself. There is a beauty queen in each of us. God put it there. All we need to do is to reach inside ourselves, and with God's help, we'll find it. Thanks for helping me to stretch my arms a little longer."

Jean has lived long — and well — enough to know that how we feel about our "station" in life really affects how we feel about ourselves. But age, or the lack of it, has little to do with how we view our "station." I wish we all were able to count our blessings as cheerfully as did my young friend Wendee Wilcox, in this uplifting theme, titled "No Wishes Left to Make," that she wrote for her second-grade class (with a little help from her father, Brad Wilcox):

Some people wish for jewelry. But I have necklaces and real clip-on earrings in my black box with light pink flowers on it. I keep my jewels on the dryer.

Many wish for money. But I have money in my milk carton in the kitchen closet. It has a "W" on it so I don't get mixed up. I'm saving for a pretty ballerina.

Lots of people wish for a house. But I have a house. It's a chicken coop, at least it used to be. It's white, but the paint is coming off. It has a slanted roof and in winter the icicles go clear to the ground if I don't knock them off. I like my bedroom best of all because the light switch is right by the door and I sleep in a warm bed that has fancy posts. It was my grandma's when she was a little girl.

Many wish for toys. But I have stuffed teddy bears. My panda is the biggest.

Some people wish for daddies and mommies. But I have a daddy and a mommy. They are good to me and teach me to never smoke or drink. My mom plays Old Maid with me and sings. My daddy wrestles with me. He reads me stories before bed and snuggles with me. If I have bad dreams I go in and sleep next to my dad. He is big, and bad dreams don't dare come to him.

Many wish for freedom. But I have freedom to not have to go to a certain church or wear certain dresses. I can make my own choices.

Lots of people wish for happiness. But I'm happy to play. I love animals and eating raspberry sherbet and singing.

Lots of people have wishes. But I already have everything they wish for. I guess I don't have any wishes left to make.

"The Station" concludes with this advice:

"So stop pacing the aisles and counting the miles. Instead, climb more mountains, go barefoot more often, swim more rivers, watch more sunsets, laugh more, cry less. Life must be lived as we go along. The final station will come soon enough."

Each year advice columnist Abigail Van Buren publishes a set of New Year's resolutions based on the original credo of Alcoholics Anonymous, with variations of her own. Here are some of her suggestions:

Just for today I will live through this day only and not set far-reaching goals to try to overcome all my problems at once. . . .

Just for today I will be happy. . . .

Just for today I will adjust myself to what is. I will face reality. I will correct those things that I can correct and accept those things I cannot correct.

Just for today I will improve my mind. . . .

Just for today I will do something positive to improve my health. . . .

Just for today I will do something I've been putting off for a long time. . . .

Just for today, before I speak I will ask myself, "Is it true? Is it kind?" and if the answer is negative, I won't say it.

Just for today I will make a conscious effort to be agreeable. I will look as good as I can, dress becomingly, talk softly, act courteously, and not interrupt when someone else is talking.

Just for today I'll not improve anybody except myself.

I'd like to add three additional resolutions of my own:

Just for today I will have a program for improvement.

Just for today I will have a quiet half-hour to relax alone.

Just for today I will be unafraid. I will gather the courage to do what is right and take responsibility for my own actions.

I learned early on that no amount of desperate dieting would take away even a quarter inch of my height (5 feet 10 inches). I had to learn to stand tall and let it work for me. The secret to feeling good about ourselves and our "station" in life is to focus on the Savior while we are improving ourselves. If we do the best we can with the gifts we have been given, He will then carry us when we are too weak to stand alone.

[1]"The Station" is reprinted from Robert J. Hastings, *A Penny's Worth of Minced Ham: Another Look at the Great Depression* (Carbondale, Ilinois: Southern Illinois University Press, 1986). All rights reserved.

10

Stop the World—I Want to Get Off!

When God was in his workshop finalizing plans for our creation, I believe he must have said, "I'll call this model Woman and give her my greatest gift—a nurturing and compassionate spirit. And I'll give her stewardship over other precious spirits." What a wonderful gift! Would you trade being a woman, the nurturer, the hub of your home? I wouldn't, and I doubt if many of us would. Even so, eons later, I wonder if Heavenly Father doesn't occasionally look down, heave a sigh, and worry that some of us have overdone a good thing.

In my opinion, there is a positive passivity—or need—that impels us to sacrifice for our loved ones when sacrifice is truly advantageous to their welfare. We all grow in the process.

But there is also a negative passivity that infringes on our rights unreasonably, causing us to become martyrs and inwardly resentful. It drains our confidence and our self-esteem and weakens those we are trying to help. Why do we act this way? Maybe we want to avoid confrontation or unpleasant situations. We want to be seen as nice. Or perhaps we don't realize there are viable alternatives.

Carol Lynn Pearson's poem "Millie's Mother's Red Dress" describes the situation perfectly. I am grateful for her permission to reprint it here:

> *It hung there in the closet*
> *While she was dying. Mother's red dress.*

97

Like a gash in the row
Of dark, old clothes
She had worn away her life in.

They had called me home,
And I knew when I saw her
She wasn't going to last.

When I saw the dress, I said,
"Why, Mother—how beautiful!
I've never seen it on you."

"I've never worn it," she slowly said.
"Sit down, Millie—I'd like to undo
A lesson or two before I go, if I can."

I sat by her bed,
And she sighed a bigger breath
Than I thought she could hold.
"Now that I'll soon be gone,
I can see some things.
Oh, I taught you good—but I taught you wrong."

"What do you mean, Mother?"

"Well—I always thought
That a good woman never takes her turn,
That she's just for doing for somebody else.
Do here, do there, always keep
Everybody else's wants tended and make sure
Yours are at the bottom of the heap.

"Maybe someday you'll get to them,
But of course you never do.
My life was like that—doing for your dad,
Doing for the boys, for your sisters, for you."

"You did—everything a mother could."

"Oh, Millie, Millie, it was no good—
For you—for him. Don't you see?
I did you the worst of wrongs.
I asked nothing—for me!

"Your father in the other room,
All stirred up and staring at the walls—
When the doctor told him, he took
It bad—came to my bed and all but shook
The life right out of me. 'You can't die,

Do you hear? What'll become of me?
What'll become of me?'
It'll be hard, all right, when I go.
He can't even find the frying pan, you know.

"And you children.
I was a free ride for everybody, everywhere.
I was the first one up and the last one down
Seven days out of the week.
I always took the toast that got burned,
And the very smallest piece of pie.
I look at how some of your brothers treat
  their wives now,
And it makes me sick, 'cause it was me
That taught it to them. And they learned,
They learned that a woman doesn't
Even exist except to give.
Why, every single penny that I could save
Went for your clothes, or your books,
Even when it wasn't necessary.
Can't even remember once when I took
Myself downtown to buy something beautiful—
For me.

"Except last year when I got that red dress.
I found I had twenty dollars
That wasn't especially spoke for.
I was on my way to pay it extra on the washer,
But somehow—I came home with this big box.
Your father really gave it to me then.
'Where you going to wear a thing like that to—
Some opera or something?'
And he was right, I guess.
I've never, except in the store,
Put on that dress.

"Oh, Millie—I always thought if you take
Nothing for yourself in this world,
You'd have it all in the next somehow.
I don't believe that anymore.
I think the Lord wants us to have something—
Here—and now.

"And I'm telling you, Millie, if some miracle
Could get me off this bed, you could look

For a different mother, 'cause I would be one.
Oh, I passed up my turn so long
I would hardly know how to take it.
But I'd learn, Millie.
I would learn!"

It hung there in the closet
While she was dying, Mother's red dress,
Like a gash in the row
Of dark, old clothes
She had worn away her life in.

Her last words to me were these:
"Do me the honor, Millie,
Of not following in my footsteps.
Promise me that."

I promised.
She caught her breath,
Then Mother took her turn
In death.[1]

I believe that there are two types of stress.

The first one is what I call the "tyranny of the urgent." This is the kind of stress that results from things over which we have no control. For instance, my husband had been ill for a year and in bed 75 percent of that time. One day I was on the phone, talking to my mother long-distance, when my husband's brother rang the bell at the front door. I could hear Hal calling from his bed, asking me to let his brother in. The cat had just thrown up on our new rug, and our two-year-old grandson was at the other end of the rug, shredding our family photo album.

At moments like these we handle the urgent, no matter the cost, and defer what is merely important to a later time. Sometimes we have no choice.

Fortunately we do have control over the second type of stress. I'll teach you a key phrase that I hope you will use when applicable and never forget. The phrase is: *"Let me be perfectly honest with you."* Here are some illustrations of how it works.

Situation 1: The husband of a working-in-the-world woman is upset. He complains that the hours she works are long and that their young son hardly knows her. She agrees. She promises that she will come home right after work that very night.

The problem arises when a colleague stops her at the office door. He says, "You've got to help me. This report is due tomorrow and I'm stuck. My job probably depends on it."

How can she turn him down? Does she stay, stomach churning, knowing her husband is fuming at home? No. There is a better way.

Situation 2: A neighbor who lives in the next block calls you one morning. She knows that you drive your children to school every day and is sure it would be no trouble at all for you to pick up her little boy and take him also. Your blood pressure soars. Your mornings are already hectic, and driving a block out of your way every day will be the last straw. What about when your own children are at home sick? Do you leave them so you can fulfill your obligation to the neighbor? Your head spins. You can't handle it, but how can you refuse? It would seem so, well, unfriendly.

Situation 3: It's late at night and you are exhausted. You pull your hands out of the dishwater and dry them off just as your daughter rushes in in her pajamas and tells you she needs five dozen cookies to take to school in the morning. She's sorry she forgot. We all know you can't allow your child to look undependable in the eyes of her teacher, so you take a deep breath, turn on the oven, and pull the ingredients out of the cabinets. Right? Wrong!

Here are suggestions on how to deal with these situations. Don't resort to negative passivity and mumble, "Oh, all right," feeling bitter and abused, or turn aggressive and scream, "No! I've put up with your inconsiderate behavior for the last time. Leave me alone!"

First of all, buy some time: "Let me get back to you." Then excuse yourself for a moment to pull your thoughts together.

Second, when you return, be kind but truthful: *"Let me be perfectly honest with you."*

Third, provide alternatives: "I can't do what you ask, but I have some other ideas for you to consider."

After excusing yourself to the business colleague at the office and spending a minute or two in the powder room, go back and say, *"Let me be perfectly honest with you.* My husband is home with our son, waiting for me. My family has to be my first priority. But I can work with you during my lunch hour tomorrow, or I have some free time Friday morning if you can arrange a slight delay for the report."

Tell the neighbor requesting a ride for her son that you'll call her back. When you call, say, *"Let me be perfectly honest with you.* I have so much going on in my life that I'm afraid I couldn't be dependable, but I'll be more than happy to pick him up in an emergency." During the interval between getting and returning the call, you might even think of another neighbor whose children are grown and for whom time hangs heavy on her hands. With a little creative effort, you may suggest someone who would welcome the chance to feel needed.

As for the cookies, you could ask, "How many do you need? Just a second. I have to check on the baby, but I'll be right back and we'll talk." When you return, tell your daughter, "Susie, *let me be perfectly honest with you.* I am exhausted. I've had a long, hard day. As I see it, you have three choices. Your father or brother can drive you to the grocery store to buy packaged cookies. Or you can make them yourself tonight, if you'd rather. Or tomorrow morning I'll drive you to the bakery, where we can pick up some of those delicious, almost homemade kinds. You decide. Good night, dear."

The best part is that the office, the neighbor, and the daughter's school will survive. And, happily, so will you.

Be careful not to judge anyone else's actions harshly, because we each walk in moccasins that are unique. One friend took me to task because I didn't agree to drive the neighbor's son to school on a permanent basis. Some women have an abundance of energy. They bake all their family's bread, sew their children's clothes, and seem to manage lots of other things that would wear most of us out. We have our own talents and stress levels, and only the woman filling the shoes knows when she is at the breaking point. Each family is individual in what it—and the wife and mother personally—can endure.

In their book *From Here to Maternity* (Bookcraft, 1987), Kathleen (Casey) Null and Carolyn Sessions Allen list ten *non*-commandments, in a tongue-in-cheek effort to expose burdens many Latter-day Saint women may be carrying around needlessly:

1. Bread-baking is not a requirement for the celestial kingdom.

2. Children in store-bought clothes will not become juvenile delinquents.

3. Quilting will not make one's calling and election sure.

4. During a temple recommend interview, the bishop does not ask sisters if they have learned to do cross-stitch.

5. Cookies and punch are not mentioned in the Word of Wisdom.

6. The consumption of TVP will not cause a sudden desire to do genealogy.

7. Making elaborate quiet books for my children may not necessarily ensure quiet.

8. Using jam from the corner store will not cause lightning to strike.

9. Putting my three-year-old in a three-piece suit and tie on Sunday will not guarantee that he'll serve a mission.

10. Plastic grapes in the living room do not keep away evil spirits.

A wise man once talked about people's ability to give and compared it to the contents of a bucket. Say you are filled to the brim at daybreak. If your supply is disbursed unchecked, you will obviously be drained by dusk. Perhaps on a scale of one to ten, you will hover at minus two. That isn't practical. You can't give what you haven't got. For your own well-being as well as the welfare of your family, you must learn responsibility for the direction of your focus.

I loved the following letter from Marilyn Gail Gilbert:

Dear Sister Barbara Jones:

I attended BYU Education Week and by some miracle got into every one of your classes. I want to thank you for enriching my life.

I am one of the seven percent of women who have never worked outside the home, and I have *always* put my husband and three kids first. The other day I got three new pairs of shoes—for *myself!* Three pairs—wow! They were on sale for $3 each. It felt great. Something new for me! I know I wouldn't have done it without you.

I have never owned a set of scriptures. After I bought the shoes, the kids and I wanted to stop at a garage sale, but I had only one dollar left. Well, we did stop, and the people had a lot of books for sale, including a triple combination and an LDS edition of the Bible. Both were in very good condition. The best part, or maybe the spirit's part, was that they were only five cents each.

Now—could you send me your makeup and hair information, and maybe something on color?

This woman understood my message perfectly. She found a way to fill her own yearnings—her bucket—without harming her family or their fragile budget.

Have you ever thought about the stress that surrounded Jesus? Crowds of men, women, and children sought Him. There were times when He was too busy or too exhausted to eat or sleep properly.

How did He exist through those years of unbelievable stress? We find the answer in Mark 1:35: "And in the morning, rising up a great while before day, he went out, and departed into a solitary place, and there prayed."

What blessings are available to each of us if only we will start and end our day with Heavenly Father, if only we will focus on the Savior and what He has taught us! Every morning I get on my knees beside my bed and say, "Father in heaven, I give you this day. I want so much to follow your will. Everything I do, I dedicate to you. Please, lead me, guide me, walk beside me. Teach me to be the wife, the mother, the teacher that you desire me to be."

Christ is the divine center of my life and my buffer against undue stress. I have given Him my day. We have formed a partnership. Whatever happens from that moment on, He and I can handle together. I pray that you too will find comfort and strength through Him.

[1]Pearson, Carol Lynn *The Growing Season* (Bookcraft, 1976), pp. 50-53. Used by permission.

11

It Takes Time to Heal

D r. Elisabeth Kubler-Ross, pioneer in the field of death and dying, alerted the medical world to the five stages of grief at the passing of a loved one. Her research indicated that dealing with each stage is necessary to the healing process. Ignoring even one stage leaves part of our psyche frozen in grief, unable to move on.

Other physicians and psychiatrists have expanded on Dr. Ross's findings, concluding that the same principle applies to a loss of any kind. Whenever one suffers a serious setback, such as death, divorce, or alienation, or sustains serious illness or injury, loses a job, or parts with something of great personal value, let's face it—pain is involved. Confidence is shattered. It takes time to heal.

My husband, Hal, recently lost his health, and to a vigorous, dynamic man, that type of loss is extremely traumatic. But because he is a strong, take-charge kind of man, he figured he could handle the feelings of inadequacy on his own. He would simply step over them and get on with his life. He was surprised to find that his frustration didn't automatically go away. Fortunately his physician recognized the problem and worked with him.

On page 107 is a chart Hal's doctor used in counseling him. Let's examine it together. When we confront major loss in any form, we begin the circle. At first we protest. We may feel disbelief, denial, shock, anger, even self-recrimination. What could we have done that we didn't do? What did we do that we shouldn't have done?

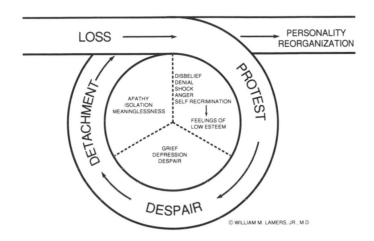

© WILLIAM M. LAMERS, JR., M.D.

Self-esteem takes a tumble. We cry profusely, and familiar patterns of sleep, eating, and digestion change markedly. Memory is often faulty.

As we begin to accept that our loss is real, despair overtakes us. Our social life is inhibited, and even our psychomotor functions (the motor effects of mental processes) are involved. We may feel grief-stricken and depressed.

When we are experiencing the protest and despair stages, we should avoid making major decisions. We need to take time to grieve and to adjust. Rosalynn Carter, in a book she wrote with her husband, former U.S. president Jimmy Carter, said that she had to grieve over her husband's disastrous 1980 defeat for the presidency of the United States before she could look to the future. She couldn't even guess at the important new roles they would fill later and that once again life would be good. *(Everything to Gain: Making the Most of the Rest of Your Life,* New York: Random House, 1987.)

In time we move from despair to a kind of *detachment,* a state in which numbness takes over, making any attempt to socialize appear overwhelming. We move through life automatically, almost zombie-like, performing daily tasks with no sense of purpose, with apathy, with feelings of isolation and meaninglessness.

But now we need to begin to try to reach outside ourselves and look for new fields to conquer.

Understanding the natural cycle is important in the coping process. When we reach that period of apathy when even hope seems dead, we need to know, at least intellectually, that we are actually on the road to recovery. We have come almost full circle, and the peace we seek is just around the next bend. We need to repeat to ourselves, "Hang in there. After the storm comes the rainbow. This too shall pass." Eventually those promises will come true, and we will move out of the circle and proceed to move forward and reorganize our lives.

Probably at no time is keeping our focus on the Savior more crucial than when we are attempting to make sense out of loss. This is the moment when bitterness, or the "Why me?" syndrome, tries to take over. This is when it is especially crucial to trust in God's perspective rather than our own.

I've asked Kris Mackay to explain why she identifies with the circle in the chart. Here is her story:

"After almost nine months of a difficult pregnancy, I delivered — and lost — a baby I desperately wanted. I have never known such despair. But realizing that my husband, Ed, and the rest of my family were suffering for me as deeply as with the sorrow of their own loss, I resolved to assist their recovery by burying my grief. I was a classic model of bravery.

"As I look back, it's scary to see how we can fool even ourselves. I was absolutely convinced I was handling my loss wonderfully until a year later, almost to the day, when I was speaking to my mother on the telephone. Without warning, my left arm began to jerk. Try as I might, I couldn't hold it still. In a matter of seconds, my leg twitched. My stomach churned. Tears poured down my cheeks. Suddenly all I could think of was the little son I had lost and how my arms ached to hold him.

"The doctor diagnosed my condition as a mild nervous breakdown. Mild? I lost weight until I looked like a skeleton loosely draped with skin. I couldn't sleep. My eyes were dark sunken holes. By burying and, in effect, denying the extent of my anguish before coming to grips with it, I had convinced myself, on the surface, that I had accepted Jon's death, leaving my battered subconscious to fight it out alone.

"For two months I couldn't concentrate to read the newspaper or watch TV. I felt constant, irrational fear. We'd moved to a new home only days before our dash to the hospital for the premature birth, so I didn't know anyone in the area. During the following year I believed I was coping well, but I see now that my ability to reach out and make new friends was definitely on hold.

"All this happened years ago, but as I look back, a couple of things stand out as if sculpted in bas-relief. One concerns a woman I barely knew. Lettie Foote is basically an introvert, but when she heard of my emotional state, she forgot about shyness and adopted me as her project. What a compassionate woman! She called and chatted on the phone, though chatting on the phone is not her style. She picked me up to go shopping. She sat by me in church. She and her husband organized a New Year's Eve party at their home, in large part, I suspect, so they could nudge my husband and me into socializing. While I was virtually catatonic with grief and couldn't have been much fun, Lettie was always there. We are still friends. I will never forget her.

"The second memory is the shock of feeling abandoned by the Spirit. Now I understand that I wasn't abandoned at all, but I was frozen in such consuming, lonely pain that I'd lost the ability to tune in to anything positive. My salvation lay in the strength of faith built up in happier times. My husband gave me a blessing every morning so I could make it out of bed, and I prayed for strength continually, in the agony of what I now perceive to be the major trial of my life.

"If you are experiencing your trial right now, let me promise you that time is a great healer. God arranged in advance for that to be so. To be sure, you never get over such a devastating loss completely, but the pain does ease. In the worst of my hurt, a doctor, a family friend, tried to comfort me by saying, 'Kris, I promise you it will get better. You will be happy again. I can't say exactly when, but you will. Hang on. It will get better.' And he was right."

My mother's experience was similar to the one Kris describes. She was close to her mother, and when Grandmother Elma developed leukemia, Mother was at her home every day, taking care of her physical needs and insisting that she look her best.

Mother has always been a strong person who taught us that you cry only over the truly big things. And sometimes not even then. Apparently she learned her own lesson too well. When Grandmother Elma died, Mother took charge. She cleaned out the house and painted it, doing in an efficient and methodical manner whatever needed to be done to settle up her mother's affairs. She didn't cry. She was too busy and too strong to give in to grief.

But one day, also a year later, Mother was driving past the cemetery where her mother was buried when she suddenly became violently ill. She pulled her car off the road and began vomiting with great wrenching gasps and weeping without restraint, in what I consider to be a physical manifestation that sorrow demands expression.

Betsy Boren suffered a different type of loss, but a loss nevertheless. Jogging in the full light of day in what she describes as "an especially safe place," she was physically attacked and brutally, senselessly beaten.

One morning, while jogging across a small bridge connecting her children's schoolyard with a family park, Betsy heard someone coming up fast behind her, striking at the fence with a stick. But she wasn't uneasy, not at all. It was a beautiful day, and the school was full of students. Besides, Betsy was and still is a kind and trusting woman. She ran in this area almost every day, and the idea of someone wishing her harm was unthinkable.

Betsy barely had time to nod to her attacker before he grabbed her and beat her without mercy. A seventeen-year-old, six-foot-six man who weighed 250 pounds, he was obviously angry at something. He struck her viciously numerous times, shattering bones in her face and arm. Then he dragged her down to the creek, tried to strangle her, and partially disrobed her in an apparent effort at rape, but abandoned her in the bushes when she lapsed into unconsciousness. In court he later admitted he had left her for dead.

Some time later a passerby heard Betsy's moans and called for help. Betsy's face was smashed beyond recognition, even to people who knew her well. They identified her by the unusual color of her sneakers. She was rushed to the hospital and into surgery, where doctors labored for five-and-a-half hours to try to reverse the damage inflicted on her and restore her shattered face. Her jaws wired shut, she lay in a coma for a month; and for another month after rousing, she had no memory. To this day some recollections of the attack are mercifully dim.

Ironically, Betsy's husband is an attorney. In a moving newspaper interview after the attack, he characterized his wife as "the kindest woman I have ever known." Yet he suffered his own excruciating loss when he stood by helplessly and watched a judge rule against trying her assailant for attempted murder. Instead, the charge was reduced to assault, a considerably less serious offense, and the man was back on the streets before his victim had barely begun to recover.

If ever there was justification for a woman to be bitter, this was such a time. Who could blame her? But Betsy's intrinsic goodness didn't allow that to happen. A stranger had robbed her of many precious things, but she didn't let him ruin her life. She recovered her sweet, trusting glow, and her smile still lights up a room. When I need a blessing from heaven, there is no one I would rather have join me in prayer.

No one lives a life totally devoid of pain. I plead with you to build up physical and spiritual strengths in advance of your trials; then trust those strengths to carry you through. Develop the habit of thinking optimistically now so that in time of need you can say, "The agony will not last forever. I am a good and worthy individual. The Lord loves me. With the help of Heavenly Father, I will endure what I must, try my very best to be the daughter he desires, and look forward to the day when once again my life will be sweet."

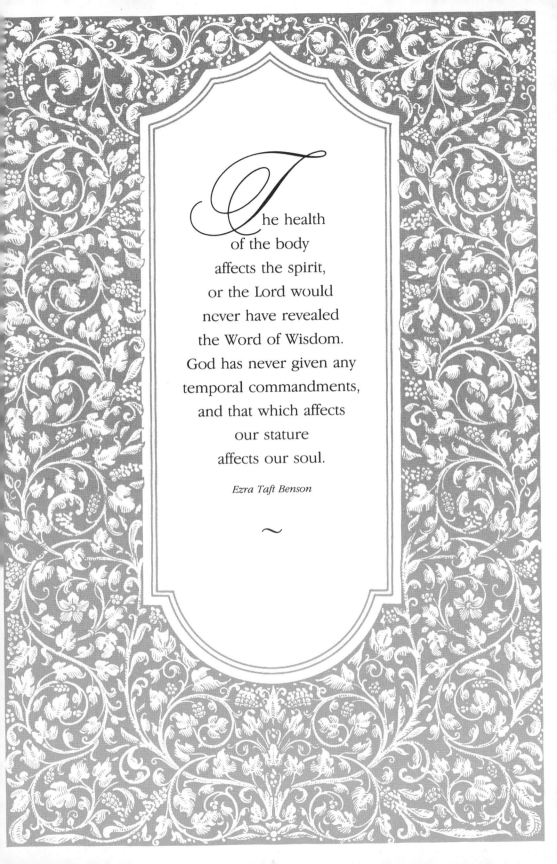

The health
of the body
affects the spirit,
or the Lord would
never have revealed
the Word of Wisdom.
God has never given any
temporal commandments,
and that which affects
our stature
affects our soul.

Ezra Taft Benson

~

12

Don't Make Food Your Friend

Brigham Young counseled: "Satisfying the appetite brings to an end the pleasure of eating; and where food is partaken of chiefly to gratify the pleasurable sensation derived from eating, disease is engendered, and true misery springs out of this gratification."

I have an interesting family, Texas born and bred. Sixty-five of my relatives live in or around El Paso, where I grew up. Uncle Bob lives in Clint, a town so small that the entering and leaving signs are virtually back-to-back. Uncle Bob is retired, and his hobby is making humorous cassette tapes. He thrives on a good joke, so I never know what will turn up in my mail. For my birthday one year he sent me an hour and a half of chirping by his canary Spot.

I have no idea where another tape came from originally, but one day while I was in Clint, Uncle Bob played what he claimed was an actual news broadcast. After four or five hilarious but questionnable "news items," the announcer broke for the following sales pitch:

"Ladies over 1,000 pounds—are you fat? Are you taller lying down than standing up? On hot days do people gather on your shady side? When you come on the scene, does the scene disappear? Is your dress size Junior Missile? Were you born on the 8th, 9th, and 10th of March? When you step on the dog's tail, do they have to call him Beaver? Is your favorite game Hide and Go Eat? When you weigh, do you go to the truck scale—and when you get off, does it go, 'Bwaaaaaaa'?

115

"If this sounds like you, you need our amazing new Flab Off. Not a liquid, not a salve, but a five-pound pill. Be sure you order the free cramming rod so you can get it down. Just send $4.95 to Clint, Texas. That's C-l-i-n-t, Clint, Texas."

I hate to tell you, but there are no free lunches. There are no magical pills. What we eat we pay for, one way or another. But we're all looking, aren't we? I told my story about Uncle Bob at a youth conference once, and from way in the back a hand shot up. "Sister Jones," came an earnest young voice from the rear, "where did you say we order that pill?"

When my daughter was thirteen years old, she ran across a full page of advertisements in a nationally-known magazine. For prices ranging from $19.95 to $25.00, magic elixirs could be purchased. One was a salve to increase chest size. Another was a mysterious substance to rub on eyelids. "Watch your eyelashes grow *overnight!*" the text promised. (I had visions of gullible teenagers parting their flowing lashes with both hands in order to see.) "Scandinavian Fat Blocker," the ad fairly screamed. "Eat and lose weight, as much as you want! No diet, no exercise! Easy and automatic! Stop counting calories! Now you can have the body you've always dreamed of!"

Let me repeat—there are no free lunches. Don't waste valuable time with gimmicks. If you know in your heart that losing weight is what you need to do and that trimming down will unlock the door leading to a more confident you, discipline is your only key.

Eat sensibly and exercise. Develop a regimen you can live with over the long haul. Stay away from fads.

Several years ago during the directors' meeting at the Miss Universe pageant, I was introduced to the group as "the body lady." I had acquired this reputation through drastic changes in the body shapes of several state winners who had trained with me. That reputation, along with my many years of ballet training, gave me the knowledge that I now share with you.

First of all, diets don't work, because they are temporary. When some women start a diet, they're geared toward thinking

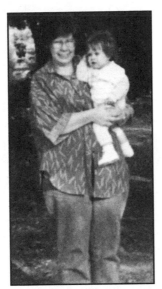 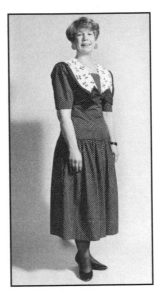

Sally Bayles, before and after diet and exercise program

they'll sacrifice, starve themselves, and be martyrs for a whole month. By that time their metabolism is so low that they gain weight back twice as quickly as they took it off, and in another month they're dieting again.

The only way to stop this miserable cycle is to find a sensible plan you can live with forever. For our purposes, let's keep it simple and easy to understand. *If you want to lose weight, cut out sugar, saturated fat, and salt.* Dairy products, such as cheese, cottage cheese, whole milk, sweetened or fruit-flavored yogurt, and ice cream contain saturated fat calories in excess. (However, women also need calcium. If an important source of your calcium is milk, drink the nonfat variety or eat nonfat yogurt or cottage cheese.) Fat calories tend to go directly to the hips and settle there. Dedicate yourself to avoiding them. What fat you need, you will get without trying.

Brigham Young was truly prophetic when he said, more than a century ago, "The Americans as a nation are killing themselves with their vices and high living. As much as a man ought to eat in half an hour, they swallow in three minutes, gulping down their food like the canine quadraped under the table, which, when a chunk of meat is thrown down to it, swallows it before you can say 'twice.' "

More good advice from Brigham Young is this: "It is crucial that you drink 8 to 10 glasses of water each day. It is difficult to find anything more healthy to drink than good cold water. This is the beverage we should drink. It should be our drink at all times."

Eat steamed vegetables, grains, and fruit, and remember to eat things the way God made them, in their natural state. Eat meat as a side dish, in small portions.

In other words, follow the Word of Wisdom, which was given by the Lord in 1833 as a guide to good health. Brigham Young explained, "To those who observe it [God] will give great wisdom and understanding, increasing health, giving strength and endurance to the faculties of their bodies and minds until they shall be full of years upon the earth. This will be their blessing if they will observe his word with a good and willing heart and in faithfulness before the Lord."

Taste is a matter of what we become accustomed to. Of course we love sauces made with sour cream and cheese, but we need to learn not to eat solely for taste. We should eat to satisfy the pangs of hunger. We need to teach ourselves to do what seems to be unnatural until it becomes second nature. In *The Road Less Traveled* (New York: Simon and Schuster, 1978), Dr. S. Scott Peck refers to this philosophy in a chapter on self-discipline. I have arranged his advice into a concise formula:

We need constant self-examination, which leads to analysis. With analysis, we find truth about ourselves. With truth comes challenge, and that means change. With challenge (and change), we know there is pain. We don't want pain, so we avoid challenge (and change).

Avoiding challenge (and change) is human nature. It is natural and easy. But being natural or easy does not necessarily mean that something is beneficial. Most of us like gravy and rich,

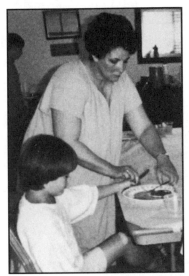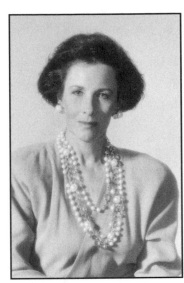

Georgina Taylor, before and after diet and exercise program

gooey additions to our food. Forgoing them may be difficult, especially in the beginning. But if our goal is to lose weight, we must teach ourselves to do what seems to us to be unnatural until it becomes second nature. And that process is called self-discipline.

We shouldn't starve ourselves, however. A starvation diet doesn't work. Instead, we should be on the alert for empty calories that we don't need. My husband says, "Train yourself not to eat solely for taste; eat to fill yourself up."

Tastes are acquired. Before long you probably will prefer nonfat milk over regular, finding that regular or whole milk has become too rich for your tastebuds. So if you are ready to eat dessert and you have the choice between a chocolate eclair and frozen nonfat yogurt, remember another of my husband's sayings: "Sometimes you have to do what you don't want to do in order to get what you want to get."

Don't let food be your friend. At least not in the negative sense. Think seriously about that phrase. Write it down and hang it on your mirror or tape it to your refrigerator door.

Do you eat only when you are hungry and your body really

needs nourishment? Or do you eat for entertainment, from lone-liness, or out of boredom? Don't let this happen. Don't snack for lack of something better to do. You undoubtedly have friends and worthwhile activities. (If not, work to enlarge that part of your life.) Think of the food that tempts you least. For me that would be stewed tomatoes. I dislike stewed tomatoes. If I were stranded on a deserted island and dying of malnutrition, I would perhaps eat stewed tomatoes. Otherwise, no. When I remember that lone brownie lurking in the freezer and feel my feet moving in that direction, I ask myself, "Are you really hungry? Would you eat a bowl of stewed tomatoes if it appeared before you now?" If my honest answer is yes, even stewed tomatoes, I know I am really hungry and that my body does need food. Even so, I would bypass the brownie and select whole-grain bread or fruit. Those foods would satisfy my craving for a much longer period and also provide me with energy.

Following are several recipes that are not only low in calories but also delicious in taste.

Barbara's Famous Power Salad

Chop finely, in equal amounts, red cabbage, broccoli, and cauliflower. Add in smaller amounts, to taste, chopped mush-rooms, grated carrot, chopped tomato, chopped red pepper, and chopped red onion. Combine vegetables. Top with a dressing made by combining low-calorie Italian and low-calorie ranch dressings.

Beauty Queens' Baked Apples

Preheat oven to 350 degrees F. Wash 6 apples. (I prefer tart green apples.) Core (don't peel) and score each apple with a knife down 1 inch from the top. Put apples in an 8-inch square baking dish. Fill center of each apple with raisins. Pour 2 12-ounce cans diet cherry soda over apples, and sprinkle with 2 teaspoons cinnamon. Bake for approximately 1 hour or until apples are very soft. Serve warm or cold. Makes 6 servings.

Pumpkin Pudding

Preheat oven to 350 degrees F. Beat lightly 2 eggs. Stir in 1 can (approximately 14 ounces) pumpkin, sugar substitute of choice to equal 1 cup of sugar, 1 teaspoon cinnamon, $\frac{1}{2}$ teaspoon ginger, $\frac{1}{4}$ teaspoon cloves, and $1\frac{1}{2}$ cups nonfat milk. Pour into an 8-inch square baking dish. Do not cover. Bake at 350 degrees for 50 minutes. Cool before serving. Makes 6 servings.

Sharlene Wells Hawkes's Prize Pasta

Cook 16 ounces (1 pound) angel hair pasta according to package directions. Heat 2 cans (14.5 ounces each) Italian stewed tomatoes and pour over cooked pasta. Sprinkle with Parmesan cheese.

Kris's No-oil, No-cholesterol, Whole Wheat Bread

Dissolve 3 tablespoons dry yeast in 2 cups warm (110 to 115 degrees F.) water; set aside until yeast is activated. Meanwhile, in a small saucepan, mix 2 cups milk, 1 rounded tablespoon salt, and 1/3 cup honey; heat to simmering point (don't boil). Then transfer it to a large mixing bowl. Add 2 cups whole wheat flour, the yeast mixture, and 2 egg whites. Beat until silky. Add 6 additional cups whole wheat flour; then gradually add 3 to 4 cups white flour until dough begins to leave the sides of the bowl.

Turn dough out onto a lightly floured board or pastry cloth. Knead dough for 10 to 15 minutes, or until it is elastic. Form dough into 3 loaves. Spray 3 bread tins with nonstick cooking spray, and place one loaf in each. Let loaves rise in pans in a warm spot for approximately $1\frac{1}{2}$ hours. Preheat oven to 350 degrees F. Bake bread on center rack for 30 to 35 minutes. It is done when the loaf has shrunk from the sides of the pan; or test by tapping bottom of the pan to release loaf, then tapping bottom of the loaf lightly. If there is a hollow sound, the loaf is done. Remove loaves from oven and cool them on wire racks.

What Will It Be — Taste or Waist?

With a little advance planning, it is possible to eat sensibly when you eat out. I love salads, but adding full-calorie salad dressings found in most restaurants will give you close to the same amount of fat as an order of french fries. Some restaurants offer low-cal dressing, but I hesitate to count on it. When I travel, I take my favorite low-calorie dressing in a small plastic bottle. I order my salad without dressing and then use my own, which I smuggle in and out of my purse.

One night when we dined at the Lido in Paris, I was attired in a black floor-length evening gown, complete with long black gloves and a jeweled, feathered cocktail hat. When my salad was served, I stealthily took my salad dressing bottle from my beaded evening bag. The maitre d' came rushing to our table, his tails flapping as he ran, and whispered in my ear, "Madame! Why are you putting hand lotion on your salad?"

Most restaurants will prepare an entrée for you without using butters and oils. Simply ask. In order not to offend the chef, you may order the sauce brought to you "on the side." You can also order your vegetables steamed and your potatoes dry. Sounds unappetizing? You have to make up your mind which is the most important to you—taste or waist.

I personally do not believe in using on a regular basis liquid-diet products such as those that come in powder form and are mixed with nonfat milk. However, they may help some individuals achieve quick weight loss and bridge the gap between heavy and more sensible eating. You should, of course, check with your doctor before embarking on any diet plan, particularly if you want to lose more than just a few pounds.

When Christina Faust, Miss California 1989, competed for the title of Miss USA 1989 in Mobile, Alabama, she was shocked to see the mounds of spaghetti and pizza being served to the contestants. Christina told me, "When you are nervous, which of course we were, you eat everything in sight, if you're not careful. I drank a glass of liquid-diet supplement in the privacy of my own room, so the edge was taken off my appetite before I faced the table of no-no's. I wouldn't advise anyone to live on liquid diets, but for a short emergency, it does usually work."

Before going to a dinner party where he knows that rich foods will be served, my husband, Hal, eats something filling and lowfat, such as a food that has complex carbohydrates, to help curb his appetite and allow him to eat sensibly.

And while we're discussing food, let me briefly mention some things doctors have recommended that women avoid if they suffer from Premenstrual Syndrome (PMS). Just before the cycle, we seem to crave sweets, especially chocolate, which contains two of the biggest PMS aggravators — caffeine and sugar. According to my gynecologist, we actually do crave sweets, and especially chocolate, due to hormonal changes. But we may make the condition worse, plummeting us into stress and depression, if we give in to those cravings. Fruits, vegetables, and grains are much more beneficial and satisfying in the long run.

Actually, we would all probably benefit if we were to reduce our intake of sugar at all times of the month. In a brochure on emotional health prepared by *Prevention* magazine, the question is asked, "How do you change a hardened criminal into a useful citizen?" The authors' answer: "Take away his candy bars." They reported on what happened when the diet of 276 teenaged boys in a Virginia detention center was altered to exclude sugar. In this "Anti-crime Diet," canned fruit was rinsed to eliminate the sugar, fruit juices and water were served instead of soft drinks, no sugar was placed on the tables at mealtimes, and no candy bars, cakes, pies, cobblers, or other sweet desserts were served. For snacks, the boys received fruit, popcorn, and celery and carrot sticks.

As a result of this sugarless menu, antisocial behavior was reduced by 48 percent, thefts by 77 percent, and assaults by 82 percent. Sugar has reportedly been curtailed in prison diets in at least forty-two states.

For our purposes, let us not forget that reduction in sugar may reward us not only with greater emotional stability, but also with weight loss.

Keeping your weight under control is important, but it is not the only thing that matters. Don't be obsessive about it. Don't let a scale be your only criterion for how you feel about yourself.

The following is from a letter written to me by Michelle Royer, Miss USA 1987:

"After I gave up my crown, I went to see Eileen Ford, who runs the Ford Modeling Agency in New York. She asked me how much I weighed, and when I told her 140 pounds, she said she couldn't use me unless I went down to 120. (I haven't weighed that since I was eleven or twelve.)

"At first I was hurt and I cried, but then I started thinking rationally. I realized I wasn't ever going to weigh 120 because I am just too tall (nearly six feet). I would look dead. I decided to throw away my scales. Now I train every day to stay healthy looking. I don't diet and I don't weigh. I do eat healthy and even splurge on chocolate every once in a while, but not too often. I feel so much better when I don't starve myself. My energy level is much higher.

"When I look in the mirror now, I see a very lucky girl. I may not have the measurements insisted upon by the modeling agency, but I am happy and healthy, and I have people in my life who are proud of me and who love me very much."

Michelle learned a valuable lesson: that true priorities in life are not dictated totally by numbers on a scale. But she also learned, as I did, that you can turn your body into something you are happy with by eating sensibly and exercising.

Some dieters fail because they overlook the fact that we human beings have a divine nature. That divine nature gives us the capacity, if we put it to use, to transform or change ourselves.

I went with my son to his first day of a New Testament class at Brigham Young University. The teacher entered the room with an armload of books, looked at the class, and asked this question: "You believe in Christ—but do you believe Christ?" Then he said, "Christ died for us, and it is through his atoning grace that we are saved."

The teacher quoted a scripture relating to grace: "If men come unto me I will show them their weakness. I give unto men weakness that they may be humble; and my grace is sufficient for all men that humble themselves before me; for if they humble themselves before me, and have faith in me, then will I make weak things become strong unto them." (Ether 12:27.)

In other words, Christ's grace takes over where our human capacity ends. He has promised that if we do our part, our very best, then He, through the power of His grace, will supply whatever we cannot handle.

Not long ago my husband was very ill with heart problems. In the middle of the night the paramedics rushed him to the hospital. As I stood by his bedside, I dreaded having to leave for a speaking engagement in another state. I told him I would cancel the engagement, but he refused to let me, saying I would do more good by helping others than by staying with him.

I didn't want to leave him, but as the last visitor left the hospital, Hal insisted it was time for me to go. For the only time I can remember, tears streamed down Hal's cheeks. I felt a lump in my throat and held back my own tears as I kissed him good-bye.

When I got into my car in the darkened parking lot, I broke down. I couldn't control the sobs any longer. I poured out my heart to my Heavenly Father: "Father, you can't take him yet. I've already survived the trauma of my first husband's death, but I couldn't live through the death of Hal."

Then in the darkness I clearly heard the still, small voice: "My grace is sufficient for thee; for my strength is made perfect in weakness." (2 Corinthians 12:9.) It was then that I felt the comfort of knowing I could handle any trial that came my way, because where I am weak, through His grace I will become strong.

The grace of Christ is available to all of us, in every needful area of our lives. He cares about what is important to us. For me in that darkened parking lot, my urgent priority was the health of my husband. For you it may be something else. Perhaps your weight is the cross you are carrying.

Please know that your answer lies with the Savior. His grace *is* sufficient for you, for His strength is made perfect in your weakness. Make Christ your partner, and you will succeed.

13

Power Walk Your Way to Health

It seems that no matter how carefully we watch the foods we eat, we don't feel at our best unless we combine sensible diet with exercise. In a conference address in the 1850s, Brigham Young commented, "My mind becomes tired, and perhaps some of yours do. If so, go and exercise your bodies." President Young understood the relationship between how we feel mentally and our physical condition, for he also said, "Let the body work with the mind, and let them both labor fairly together, and with but few exceptions, you will have a strong-minded, athletic individual, powerful both physically and mentally.

A lot has been said and written about a body's "set point." The basic philosophy behind this idea is that each body has a certain point, a particular weight, that is based on caloric intake and activity, and no matter how many pounds we might lose on a crash diet, we eventually go back to that weight. The only way to keep the pounds off is to lower our set point through exercise. Regular exercise makes our metabolic rate — the rate at which we burn calories — go up, and that increases our ability to lose weight.

Other benefits of regular exercise are that we become healthier because the heart works harder, and a strong heart pumps more blood with less effort; our blood-sugar level remains stable, because the muscles use more fat than sugar as fuel; and food passes more rapidly and easily through the digestive tract.

We also feel better when we exercise because exercise releases into the brain endorphins, which are natural, nonaddictive, morphinelike painkillers. Endorphins contribute to a jogger's heightened ability to withstand pain while running. One group of joggers could withstand deliberately inflicted pain about 70 percent longer after running a mile than they could before running. Endorphins also have been found to affect moods, possibly contributing to the "runner's high" that people feel at the end of a long, grueling run. Watch for the sense of well-being you experience after any consistent, vigorous exertion.

But running takes its toll on knee and ankle joints. Personally, I prefer fast walking. And remember that walking for fitness is not the same thing as strolling. Here are some suggestions to help you start your walking regimen.

First, put on your exercise clothing, including good-quality running shoes. Next, put on a headset battery-operated tape player with a tape of your favorite music; this will occupy your thoughts while you time your exercise period. Then start walking . . . *power walking.*

Use a heel-toe, heel-toe, heel-toe motion. Stand erect, tuck your hips under, and walk with power. With elbows bent, pump your arms as you stride. Arm action helps to increase walking speed and to trim the waistline. For additional benefits, carry two-pound or three-pound weights. Stride with conviction, your pace as brisk as possible. To get a good workout, speed walk for approximately forty-five minutes at least five days a week. If you listen to a forty-five-minute tape, listen to marches or other upbeat music and walk until your tape needs turning over; then walk back.

A treadmill is an excellent exercise machine if you can afford one, because it is available at any hour, in the safety of your own home. Try it out in the store before you purchase it.

Whether you walk outdoors (this is preferable) or on a treadmill indoors, as your muscles grow stronger and your heart rate improves, your speed and distance will increase. It is important to do stretches both before and after walking, to minimize aches and pains. (See illustrations, pages 128–131.)

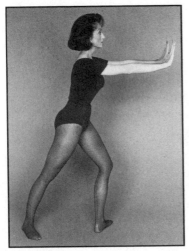
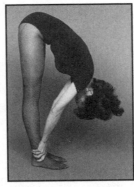
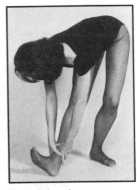

Calf stretch: (Above left) Stand at arm's length away from a wall. With hands pressed against wall and left knee bent, stretch right leg back, keeping heel on floor. Hold for 20 seconds. Change legs and repeat. *Back-of-leg stretches:* (Center) Stand with feet together. Bend forward and grasp ankles: hold for 20 seconds. Bend knees and roll up. Do this three times. (Right) While standing, bend back leg and stretch front leg forward and flex. Bend forward with hands holding on to ankles and try to "kiss" your toe. Hold for 10 seconds; then repeat on opposite side. Do this four times.

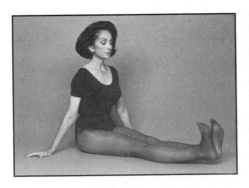
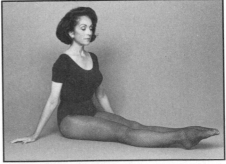

Ankle flex and back-of-leg stretch: Flex the feet (above left). Then point the toes (above right). Do this ten times. Next, gently bend forward, trying to touch your nose to your knees (right). Do not force this motion or bounce. Hold for 20 seconds. Do this four times.

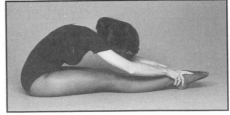

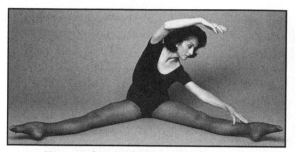 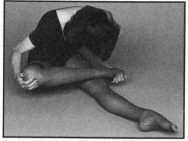

Torso and inner thigh stretch: (Above left) Sit on floor with back straight, legs stretched out to sides. Stretch toward left leg, bringing right arm over head. Hold for 15 seconds. Stretch to other side. Do this four times. *Stretching ham strings (back thigh muscles).* (Above right) Sit on floor with legs stretched out in front of you. Bend right knee and place right ankle on top of left knee. Holding onto right foot, bend upper body forward and hold for 15 seconds. Raise upper body. Switch legs and repeat stretch. Do this two times.

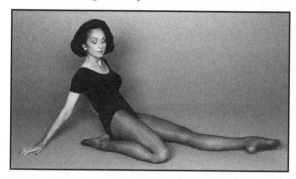

Stretching front of thigh: (Left) With legs in parallel position, bend right leg to outside of thigh. Gently lean back, using arms as support (do not force this motion). Hold for 20 seconds. Take leg back gently. Then repeat on left side. Repeat. Do this two times.

There are other advantages to exercise. Here are excerpts from three letters written by Bonniejean Gatten of Las Vegas. Notice her change in attitude from the first letter to the last.

Letter #1: "Thank you so much for coming to Las Vegas. . . . I am 45, a single parent, and moved to Las Vegas a year ago. When I hear the statistics about the ratio of women to men in the Church, it is a struggle to maintain a positive outlook. I know my chances of remarrying in this life are slim. I know that my weight decreases my attractiveness, but worst of all it lowers my self-esteem.

"You have inspired me to try once and for all to get the weight off and keep it off. Surely gluttony and other incorrect eating habits are not in conformity with the spirit of the Word of Wisdom. So you see why I hung on every word you spoke. You are a saleswoman of hope!

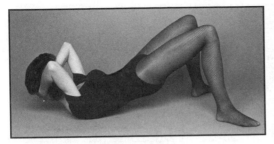

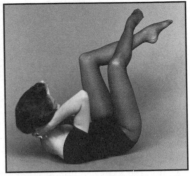

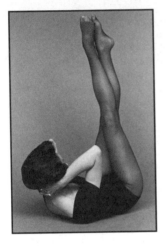

Stomach tighteners: (Above left) Lie on your back with legs stretched out and hands behind head. Bend legs, then lift buttocks out without straining lower back. Then gently "crunch" forward, trying to reach your nose to your stomach. Start with 10 crunches (goal is approximately 50). (Left) Lie on back with legs stretched out and hands behind head. Raise legs to 90-degree angle with legs crossed at ankles. With hands still behind head, gently press forward, raising shoulders off the floor. While in this position, "crunch" gently forward, as if trying to touch nose to knees, 10 times; then release. Repeat 10 times (trying to eventually do stretch with as few releases as possible). (Above right) Do same exercise with legs bent.

"I want to be the beautiful daughter Heavenly Father planned for me to be, but I feel I have let Him down in that department. But even if it is not meant for me to marry during this life, at least I will be peaceful, knowing I have made every effort to make myself into the person He wants me to be."

Letter #2: "You may not remember me. I attended your workshops when you were in Las Vegas last year and wrote to you, and you asked me to keep you posted. As of last December, I had lost 40 pounds, mainly from walking. As I walked, I was inspired to think about Christina Faust's talk when she came here with you and how her mother would say, 'Have faith in yourself. God has a plan for you.'

"I got up to walking five miles a day in the summer and two-and-a-half when I teach during the school year. I was maintaining

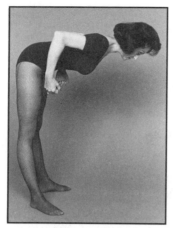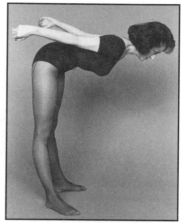

Upper arm tightener: Begin with arms at 90-degree angle (left). Stretch arms straight back (right); hold for 30 seconds; then release and return to 90-degree angle. Do this 20 times. (This exercise can also be done without bending elbows, or with two-pound weights.)

my weight loss until December, when I slid backwards. Dear friend, any pearls of wisdom would be welcome right now, as I struggle to take it a day at a time." (I sent to Bonnie some information on diet and power walking.)

Letter #3: "Here is another success story you can add to your list. . . . You are responsible in large measure for my recent marriage to Charles Michael Reinhart. Thanks to your inspiring talks, I began to have confidence in myself. I continued to work on improving my self-esteem by losing weight, walking, and reading the scriptures and other inspiring literature. (Remember — I had been single for ten years and had lost hope.)

"I dated an interesting man for two years, and it was a thrill that he even asked me out. But on March 10, Charlie asked me out for the first time. He had been baptized in January, and I met him a week later. We had a whirlwind romance and were married last Tuesday, April 24, by my bishop. We plan to be sealed in the temple early next year. I'll send you an invitation!"

How exciting it is for me to read letters like these and to picture the amazing changes in lives when commonsense principles are practiced. Another letter moved me deeply. The writer

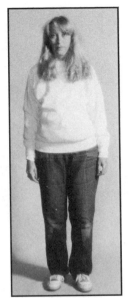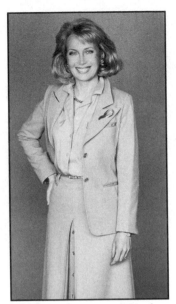

Jean Joseph, a power walker, started by walking to mailbox, then
increased distance (see page 8). Her story inspired Cindy Wilson

has gone through unbelievably heavy trials and expresses her
gratitude for exercise:

"Exercise gives you a grasp on success. You have willed yourself to accomplish something, and each day you go a little further.
It is the one time during a day full of tears and the same desert
of nothingness that you are free to push through the maze. Though
your conscious mind knows agony, the subconscious can still be
fed.

"I truly believe it is one's ability to never give up, to never
accept defeat, to believe in tomorrow and press on, that divides
survivors from quitters. Most people can stay motivated for two
or three months; a few can last for two or three years. But a
winner stays motivated for as long as it takes to win. If you don't
care where you are going, any road will take you there. But when
every conceivable avenue has been exhausted, God will pick you
up and help you find the way.

"My problem was that at age eleven, I was thrust into a pit
of darkness so horrible and totally incomprehensible that it was

as if another head had been tied onto mine. My ability to reason, think, remember, and act were normal, but my emotional system was suddenly frozen in hell. It was all I could do to drag myself out of bed and to school, where I had another set of problems.

"My father was the music teacher in a small rural community. The students thought he was too strict, so they took out their anger on me. They poured water on my head in the restroom, filled my locker with garbage so it spilled out onto the floor, called me names, and spit at me in the lunch line. I had no friends. I went through the motions of living, but I felt dead.

"I didn't confide in my parents. I believed if they knew how mixed up I was, they wouldn't love me. I worried that even God would hate such an obviously despicable person — until I received a patriarchal blessing at sixteen. I approached the patriarch with great fear and trembling, certain he would put his hands on my head and there would be no blessing for me. When he pronounced the words, it was as though the Lord Himself came down and threw His arms around me. Tears spilled down my cheeks. In that brief moment, my first shred of joy appeared. I knew God loved me. I knew He had a purpose for me. I knew I would survive.

"Nevertheless, my trials weren't over. Added to my emotional trauma, physical ailments continued to plague me. At one point I begged God to let me die. I walked out in front of a semitrailer. The driver slammed on his brakes, honked his horn angrily, and my life, such as it was, was spared.

"Back in the fifties, medicine hadn't done much with mental health. I was terrified they'd lock me up and give me shock treatments. I finally went to a doctor who gave me tranquilizers, said I'd had a nervous breakdown, and sent me home. Now that my parents realized I was troubled, they gave me a rundown on the mental illness that runs in our family. The tranquilizers helped, and I eventually married and began a family. My baby was a few months old when I was taken with rheumatic fever. The doctor told me I would never again live a physically normal life, but I recalled the power I'd felt at the time of my blessing and determined never to give up. I pushed the baby in his buggy, a short distance at first, then five miles, uphill, to my mother's. A few years and several miscarriages later (not caused by the exercise), I delivered a second baby, and then another. Altogether, my husband and I had four children. Life was a constant struggle against despair.

"In 1969 I heard Dr. Kenneth Cooper speak on aerobics in the Salt Lake Tabernacle. What a thrill! Not only was exercise good for me, but he said it created wonderful little things called endorphins, homemade tonics made by the body that did wonders for depression. As the years went by, I would strap one child to a bike, put another in a pack on my back, lift the other two onto their own bikes, and away we'd go. I was finally living.

"Then my darling little Angie developed leukemia. President Spencer W. Kimball was visiting the hospital, so her nurse asked him to come to her room. He did. My husband assisted the prophet in giving our daughter a blessing wherein President Kimball promised that she had filled her earthly requirements. He said it was time for her to go home.

"Two weeks later, on a snowy evening in December 1980, I knew it was time for Angie to leave. I requested that everyone else step out of the room. I took that frail little body in my arms and held her for the last time. I thanked God for lending her to us and committed her into His care and keeping. Suddenly the room was filled with brightness. I realized that death is like opening a door to another room so beautiful and glorious that to feel sorrow on such an occasion would be out-of-place.

"But depression or, as I eventually learned, my inherited chemical imbalance, still haunted me, in spite of new and helpful medication. I decided to really test the exercise theory and give those endorphins a real try. I joined a gym and began an intensive workout program. I wanted desperately to get off my medicine, fearful of its side effects. It was difficult at first, but my strength increased, and I began to feel wonderfully positive feelings. I slept like a brand new puppy dog. I started to cut down on

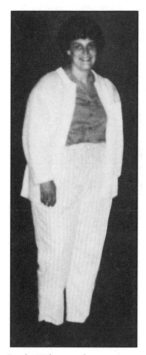 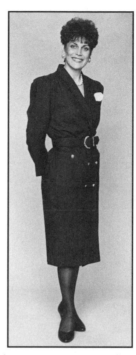

Cindy Wilson, whose story is told in chapter 1, is a power walker.

medication and have been off it entirely for the past eight years. At the age of fifty, I run, lift weights, and do aerobics.

"Life is good now and I have learned to my delight that there are things to enjoy. If your soul is in torment, as mine was, and life seems empty, fill it with beautiful things. Play soothing music. Check out lovely pictures from the library. Read uplifting books. Visit museums. Fill your home with flowers. Do something to help someone else; there are so many other people in need. Lean on the Lord. Talk to Him when you walk, run, do dishes, pull weeds. Give Him a ring; He'll never hang up on you.

"Well, Barbara, this has been a long letter. Let me close with what I tell anyone I know who suffers from depression: Place a picture in your mind of where you wish to be, a peaceful, tranquil scene. Go to that scene often, and believe that person can be you. If you believe it with all your might—and work to bring it about—it will happen!"

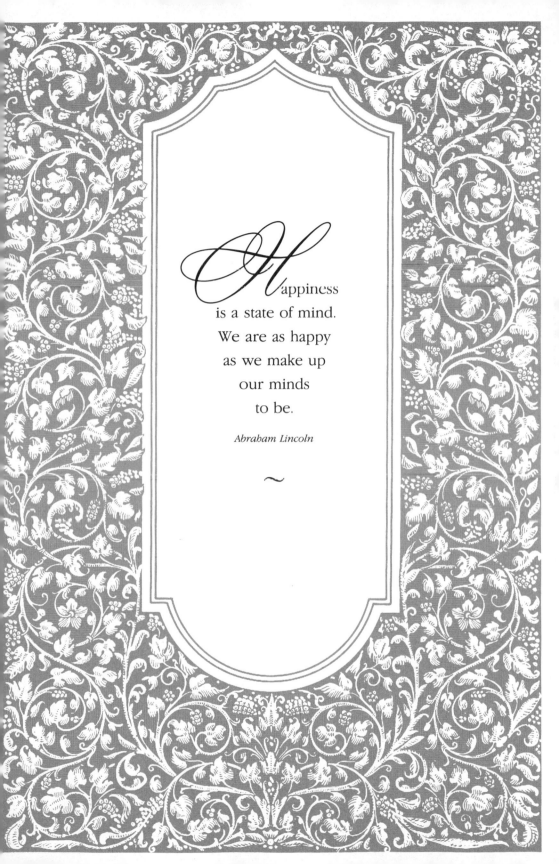

*H*appiness
is a state of mind.
We are as happy
as we make up
our minds
to be.

Abraham Lincoln

~

14

Develop a Sense of Humor

There is power in humor. If you can make someone laugh —
or, more important, if you can laugh together — life develops
a glow. Valuable lessons are learned more easily. Problems seem
less frightening. There are documented cases where people with
serious illnesses have laughed themselves back to health. A good
sense of humor is vital to the poise and well-being of the confident
woman.

Believe it or not, humor can be developed. I am living proof
of that fact. In the midst of a weekend that I perceived to be one
of the most frustrating of my life, I learned three things:

1. We have to look for the humor in our lives. (Sometimes
we have to look pretty hard.)

2. We have to be willing to laugh at ourselves.

3. After we have found the humor in unpleasant situations,
we have to use it to our advantage.

I haven't always appreciated the value of a good chuckle. Our
house was quiet and orderly while I was growing up, since I was
an only child for my first ten years. My father was an accountant,
and my mother taught etiquette in a private girls' school. Conduct
was all-important. Decorum was the watchword in our home.

Most people have an instinctive love for the lighter side. They
relate to humor. I did not. I was extremely introverted, not popular at all, and I was so tall and long-legged that kids called me
Spider. My goal was to become a classical ballerina. I practiced
ballet from the time I was five years old.

And I made it! I became a professional dancer. Now I work

139

with beauty queens. It was exciting to help train five Miss USAs in a row through my association with Guyrex Associates and to hear the announcer's voice boom out five times, "And the winner is . . . ," — and to hear each time the name of one of the young women I had helped coach. By the fourth win, even oddsmakers were publishing odds against its happening again.

When I was growing up, I promised myself I would never be an etiquette teacher like my mother; I wouldn't do that to my children. So what did I do? I managed two modeling schools. Ingrained habits are hard to break, and I raised John and Wendy with my own brand of total etiquette.

The thing I knew I could never be was a speaker. When it was my turn to read aloud in the third grade, I sniffled and froze. It went that way all through high school. In my senior year, tears streamed down my cheeks while I was presenting an oral book report; my knees shook and my voice quivered.

Soon afterwards I won a Miss America preliminary in my hometown in Texas. Sounds impressive, doesn't it? To be honest, I was Miss El Paso, and there were only eleven young women in the pageant. But I did win the title, exept that I don't remember making many appearances that year — maybe one or two. Then the year was over, and it was time to relinquish my crown. I stood in front of the townspeople and sobbed. Giving up the crown was not what brought on my tears; it was the attempt to say a few words in public. My mother was really embarrassed.

With this background, I was shocked when Brigham Young University called a few years ago to invite me to be a youth speaker. As a recent convert, I didn't understand what a youth speaker was. I didn't know what one looked like. I called my mother, and her response was short and to the point: "Well, I hope you told them you can't speak."

My first assignment was to speak at a youth conference, and if I was hazy about what a youth speaker was, I was totally in the dark about youth conferences. I went wearing my big black straw hat (I wore a hat everywhere, of course) and my fashionable black-and-white checked suit. I was total etiquette personified.

The whole weekend was a nightmare. The young people poured into the classroom wearing jeans and speaking a language I simply didn't comprehend. I stood in front of them with great decorum, my hat still on, and said sweetly, "Take out your scriptures, class, and turn to Proverbs, chapter three, verses five and six." They tuned me out after one glance, and I did nothing to change their minds. To those teenagers on that day, I was a living sleeping pill.

I couldn't believe this was happening to me. I looked up in despair and thought, *Heavenly Father, you have made a big mistake if you think I can fit in here!*

That night I went to the dance. I had been assured during my interview that all speakers dance with the young people, but I couldn't imagine anyone there asking me to dance. Brad Wilcox, one of the other speakers, saw me standing around feeling awkward and out-of-place, as I had all through school. He picked out a good-looking young man with a crew cut, maneuvered him in my direction, and said, "David, why don't you ask Sister Jones to dance?" "Brother Wilcox," David replied with a wince, "my leg is killing me!"

But the worst blow came when a sweet eighteen-year-old girl stood up in testimony meeting Sunday morning and, sniffling just as I used to, said, "I want to th-thank Sister Jones for taking the time to t-talk to me last night. I really feel c-close to her, even though (sniff) she *is* four times my age." That made me seventy-two, and the worst part is that I guess I acted that age.

As the weekend mercifully drew to a close, I shared my dismay with Brad. Through clenched teeth I said, "This is my first youth conference and my last. I'll never do this again. I mean it!" Brad coaxed, "Barbara, don't look at it like that. Try to remember back to when you were their age. Think of humorous experiences in your own early life that youth can relate to." That was some of the best advice I ever received. Thinking about what I'd seen Brad and Clark Smith, one of the other youth speakers, accomplish at the conference through their occasional use of humor, I grasped for the first time that wise words are swallowed and digested with much more relish when coated with the sweetness of humor. That advice applies not just to young people. I see now that all of life is more fun when it is taken without such deadly seriousness,

As I thought back to my childhood, lo and behold, some of the worst of times were funny when viewed through the passage of years. I grew to my present awesome five-foot-ten-inch height, barefoot and with my hair mashed down flat, between fifth and sixth grades. I remember loping along the halls at school, concentrating, just trying to keep my arms and legs going in the same direction, with all those little boys running around down by my ankles. I did have one good friend through high school, exactly my same size, and we were called the Bobbsey Twins. I remember her saying, "If one more little boy asks me how the weather is up here, I'm going to tell him it's raining and spit on his head!"

When our Civic Ballet Company performed *The Sorcerer's Apprentice,* guess what role I danced? Yes, it was a solo—as the lead broom. And when I was in *Hansel and Gretel*, did I get to be the witch? No such luck. With my height, I was relegated to being Hansel.

These things were excruciating at the time but are funny in retrospect, and sharing them lets young people know that whatever pain they are experiencing, I understand. I've been there. It will pass.

I have lightened up considerably, and now the teenagers and I relate. At a subsequent conference, the girls talked me into performing at a talent show, in front of twelve hundred young men and women, doing an act that they devised for me. It had something to do with peeling and eating a banana very dramatically, to the strains of the theme from *2001—A Space Odyssey*. Printed words can't do the skit justice, so suffice it to say that I was a hit. The teens stood up and cheered. As for my reaction, again I was close to tears, but this time it was different. I sniffled, "They liked me. *They liked me!*"

I am finally learning to have fun by looking for the humor in life, laughing at myself, and, most definitely, finding the humor in unpleasant situations. But what about you? Don't you love to be around positive, happy people, especially people who can make you laugh? How can you develop a sense of humor?

For some, making others laugh is a natural gift, but I know that it is a gift that can be developed. First you need to start looking for the humor in your life. Buy a special notebook just for this purpose, keep it handy, and write down everything that is humorous to you. The key is to write it down.

I write down in a section of my planner everything that happens to me that I find humorous. For example, at a young women's conference in Amarillo, Texas, where I once spoke, a thirteen-year-old girl got up to bear her testimony and said, "I just want to thank Suzy for lending me her slip so I could come up here today." Smiling, I wrote it down.

In a general conference session, President Thomas S. Monson told of a letter President Ezra Taft Benson had received after heart surgery. The letter said, "Dear President Benson, I know that you will be blessed for this surgery because in the Bible it says 'blessed are the pacemakers.' " With a smile, I wrote this down.

That evening we had dinner with Elder and Sister Robert E. Wells. Elder Wells told us about another General Authority who, after a heart attack, had had to have bypass surgery. A second-grader sent him a handmade get-well card. On the front the child drew a picture of a long, black rectangular box, representing a coffin, with a lone flower poking out the center. Inside he printed in big letters, "HOPE YOU GET WELL SOON, BUT IF NOT, HAVE FUN." I laughed heartily, then wrote it down.

Buy some books on humor or humorous subjects. Many are available in bookstores. I recently purchased one titled *Children's Letters to God*, compiled by Stuart Hample and Eric Marshall (New York: Workman, 1991). Here are sample letters that I wrote down in my planner:

"Dear God, on Halloween I am going to wear a Devils Costume. Is that all right with you? Marnie."

"Dear God, Do animals use you or is there somebody else for them? Nancy."

"Dear God, Maybe Cain and Abel would not kill each other so much if they had their own rooms. It works with my brother. Larry."

When my husband, Hal, came home from work that evening, I couldn't wait to read some of these humorous letters to him. I was pleasantly surprised when he took out of his wallet a piece of paper on which he had written down the following anecdote, titled "Hard to Swallow":

"The vet prescribed daily tablets for our geriatric cat, Tigger, and after several battles my husband devised a way to give her the medication. It involved wrapping Tigger in a towel, trapping her between his knees, forcing her mouth open, and depositing the pill on the back of her tongue. David was proud of his re-sourcefulness until one hectic session when he lost control of both cat and medicine. Tigger leaped out of his grasp, paused to inspect the tablet — which rolled across the floor — and then ate it."

I laughed — and wrote it down.

At a Thanksgiving family reunion in Texas, my Aunt Becky asked my Uncle Bob, "Will you love me when I'm old and gray?" He replied, "I'll not only love you, but I'll write to you wherever you are." At dinner that night Bob told Hal, "When Barbara was a teenager, she was built just like a two-by-four. If it wasn't for the lump in her throat, she wouldn't have had any shape at all. She was so tall, even back then, that she could hunt geese with a rake." I laughed — and wrote it down on my napkin, to be transferred to my planner later.

As she was chauffering me around Phoenix, where I spoke at a conference, a seventeen-year-old girl told me that when she gets married, she is going to give her children unusual names, like those of her two best friends — Betty Batty and Shirley Turley. "For instance," she said, "if I marry a man named Frisbee, I'll name my son Chase A. Frisbee. If I marry a man named Surface, I'll name my children Rocky and Sandy. And if I marry a man named Lee, I'll name my daughter Sara and my son Brock." I laughed — and wrote it down.

Now, you never know when all the humorous things you have

written down in your notebook will come in handy. With your newly developing sense of humor, you'll have opportunities to make someone laugh.

For example, when I went to my doctor's laboratory for a series of blood tests, I wrote my name down for the secretary and we started to talk about names. I opened my planner and shared with her my conversation with the young woman in Phoenix, and soon the whole office was laughing. As I left, one of the staff commented, "You're so funny, please come again You really brightened my day." Me, funny? Well, hardly, but I'm trying.

Now, it isn't that I have any aspirations to be a comedian; it's just that people don't expect a regular lay-person like you or me to come out with jokes or funny one-liners. And because of this, we can be perceived as really funny. People love to laugh, and when we make others laugh, it feels like they have wrapped their arms around us. Each of us can form new friendships stamped and sealed with humor, and we ourselves will have a lot of fun while spreading a little laughter.

There isn't a person in the world who doesn't have something to weep over. The trick is to make the laughs outweigh the tears. So I want to challenge you to work on developing your sense of humor. Buy a notebook and start writing in it. Then, when your family starts laughing at some of your newly developing, sometimes corny, humor, get them involved also and watch them grow together with the power of humor.

15

There Was a King Once . . .

There was a king once, but nobody suspected he was of royal blood because he traveled in disguise. He didn't fault his subjects for not knowing him by sight. Looking into the mirror, he barely recognized himself. Then one day he met a beautiful princess . . .

Improving oneself is not strictly a woman's prerogative.

Darwin Nimer was twenty-eight years old and had never asked a woman for a date. Maybe one of them would have accepted. He didn't know. The problem was that he was uncomfortable with himself—how he looked, how he dressed, his personality, his ability to put together an interesting evening for an interesting woman.

It wasn't that women weren't nice enough to him. Nobody was unkind. It was just that during high school his weight had ballooned up to 276 pounds, and he felt that he couldn't inflict himself on the kind of woman he wanted to ask out. With strict standards concerning the person he hoped to marry—someday— he couldn't bring himself to offer any less to her.

Darwin worked as a custodian in a church building near my home in northern California. Sometimes I take my clients to that church to use the stage, as they learn to walk and move about gracefully. Occasionally I have seen him pause at the door, listening to my instructions and enjoying the music.

One day, like the king in the fairy tale, Darwin decided it was

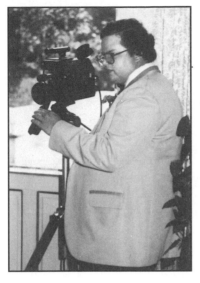
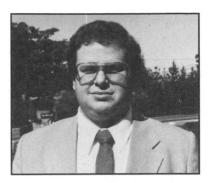

Darwin Nimer before
his transformation

time to peel out of his disguise. He watched what he ate. He exercised. He lost about seventy pounds.

Then, in the reception line at his sister's wedding, he stood next to the most beautiful woman he had ever seen. A princess! Actually, he had known her slightly from the past, but she had been away, studying at Brigham Young University. They talked for hours, and for him, at least, it was a wondrous night filled with magic.

When she told him she was headed back to school the following week but would return in three months, he was almost grateful she would be gone. He needed that time to prepare.

The next night he rang my doorbell at home. "Barbara," he said wistfully, "I've met the most wonderful woman named Trisha. I want to marry her, but there's no way she'd even go out with me. I don't dare approach her. I've seen firsthand what you do for women. I've seen the doors that open for them. So I want to ask you"—here he gulped and kicked at a pebble with his toe—"is it possible that what you do could work for me? I'm a man, but would you consider me crazy if I asked you to do my colors and to help me decide what clothes I should wear?"

He was so earnest that my heart went out to him. I said, "Let's go for it!" and from that evening on, the two of us embarked on a lengthy but almost scientific search for the real King Darwin.

Over the next few months he spent a lot of time in my family room, asking questions. "What would be a fun evening? Where should we go for a drive? If we're out to dinner and the maitre d' pulls out her chair, where should I stand? How should we order? How does your husband do it?" He wanted polish — not to become Miss USA, of course, but to woo and win his one true love.

When Trisha broke her foot, he sent a get-well card. He went regularly to young-adult activities; he needed practice in talking with women. Finally, when Trisha came home with plans for a mission in six months, he asked her out to dinner with friends.

Darwin dreamed of a day-long date. We spent one whole evening planning it in detail. The morning of the date, when Trisha thought she had been invited to breakfast on cheesecake and orange juice at the airport, he dangled four envelopes before her eyes. Inside were four keys, unlocking four cars, each a different model, waiting for them at the Los Angeles airport, for he had decided to take her to southern California for a day. Her choice of automobile would transport them from the plane to their fantasy date at Disneyland.

Another time he invited her to a movie but slipped away the evening before to watch it by himself. He had to be certain it was a movie she would enjoy. When an actor used a word he didn't understand, he raced home to look it up in the dictionary. If she happened to inquire, the explanation could fall trippingly from his tongue. On Valentine's day he sent her six lovely red roses. (The other six he kindly sent to me.)

Darwin spent a lot of time on his knees, asking the Lord for guidance. Did he have the right to ask Trisha to marry him when she was planning a mission? Meanwhile, she prepared and submitted her mission papers. Usually a prospective missionary receives the call in about ten days. After three weeks, she still hadn't received hers.

One night Darwin blurted out in desperation, "Trisha, are

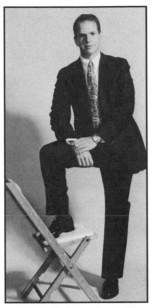 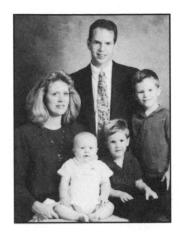

Darwin Nimer today (left), and with his wife, Trisha, and three sons

you going to marry me, or what?" Astonished, she replied, "You've never asked me!" So he did ask—and Trisha said yes. When they counseled with their stake president, he said, "Great! Don't worry about Trish's missionary papers. I'll call Salt Lake to stop them."

Was their marriage really the will of the Lord, as Darwin believes? Apparently so. The stake president called the missionary department in Salt Lake City and learned that Trisha's papers had been unaccountably misplaced.

All that took place seven years ago, and Darwin has never reverted. He is determined to remain the man his wife learned to love. Every nine months or so he notices a few pounds creeping up on him, but with a couple of weeks of special care—eating an egg and unbuttered toast for breakfast, half a grapefruit at ten o'clock, a baked chicken breast with crackers and salsa for lunch, and an apple at night—the pounds melt off again. When he changed jobs, he decided to take one that required even more exertion. For Darwin, his resolve to change permanently is well worth the effort.

There was a king once . . . and now Darwin's kingdom consists of his beloved Trisha and their three small sons.

One final note: In the delicate balance of husband-and-wife relations versus the difficult act of change, ideally the goal of self-improvement is to feel comfortable with how one looks. Only then are we free to forget our appearance and reach out to those we love.

One pitfall is that a spouse may initially interpret change, even change for the better, as a threat. To one who is at ease with the status quo, the unknown can be frightening. How deep will the change go? Will it affect the relationship? And the bottom line is, Will he (or she) still need me? One afternoon Cindy, the queen in chapter one, was surprised to discover her husband shedding a few nervous tears in the cornfield, when he thought he was alone. After he was reassured of her love, the insecurity didn't last.

We must be supportive of each other—wives of their husbands, and husbands of their wives. The ability to love is perhaps the greatest gift of life. At times of change, we must make it lovingly clear that alterations on the outside do not alter the contours of the heart.

16

Choose Your Heroes with Care

We sometimes tend to take on the personality traits and may even come to resemble those we admire. If you wish to be truly beautiful in every sense of the word, choose your heroes with care.

I have already described certain aspects of my life. Now let me approach the same situations from a different angle.

There have been many people in my life whom I have looked up to, people who, so to speak, have been my heroes. When I studied with the New York City Ballet, I put the school's prima ballerina on a pedestal and thought of her as everything I hoped to become. She was beautiful, a breathtaking dancer, and thin. I wanted to be just like her.

Everybody around me was consumed with losing weight so, of course, I was too. I starved myself until I got thinner and thinner and then so anemic and sick that eventually I had to go home. I was convinced that the dream of my life was over.

It wasn't until I read the book *Dancing on My Grave*, an autobiography written by ballerina Gelsey Kirkland with her husband, Greg Lawrence, that I knew that the ballerina I had tried so hard to emulate, my heroine, was in reality a drug addict. In order to withstand the pain and have inhuman endurance and stamina, she had turned to cocaine.

Then I went to the University of Arizona for a year. My roommate was gorgeous, with red hair, a tall, perfect figure, and the most beautiful legs I had ever seen. She was very popular on campus, and again I said to myself, "She's my hero. She's everything I could ever hope to be." But it wasn't long before I found her smoking marijuana in our dorm. I was horrified, but she was popular and I was not. Maybe she was right. Maybe I was the one who needed to change. I couldn't help but wonder.

I returned home from college and resumed my friendship with a boy I had dated all through high school. I thought he was everything I had ever wanted in a man. Even today, speaking his name strikes a chord in my heart. I will never forget him. But I remember a passage from Tennessee Williams's play *A Streetcar Named Desire*. It describes a boy who had a nervousness, a tenderness, about him that didn't ring true, a softness that wasn't quite like a man, though he was not effeminate-looking in the least. Those words described my hero.

Then we became engaged and sent out the invitations. Our wedding was a week away. But he didn't act like a typical, eager bridegroom-to-be. He didn't look me in the eye, didn't touch me or kiss me goodnight, and he was drinking constantly. Then one night he went to a local bar and became drunk and violent. After he began smashing with a baseball bat the windshields of cars parked on the street outside the bar, he was taken to jail. The young man I had loved for years and was prepared to trust with my life wasn't my hero, after all. Do you know how long I cried and still feel traces of that pain inside me?

So I married his best friend. I didn't love him as I had loved my former fiancé, but all my friends were married, and I was psychologically ready for a new hero.

But this man turned out to be a manic-depressive. Once I found him unconscious on the bathroom floor after he had taken a megadose of aspirin tablets, and he had to be rushed to the hospital to have his stomach pumped. Another time, he took all my scrapbooks out to the backyard and burned them. It had taken me a lifetime to put the books together, and they were irreplaceable.

Three times he tried to kill me with a loaded gun, and three times I cried out to my Heavenly Father, and He was there for me.

Who is *your* ultimate hero? Who will never let *you* down? Whom do *you* wish to be like?

You'll never find a better hero than Jesus Christ. Let me join Alma in asking, "Have you received his image in your countenance? Have you experienced this mighty change in your heart?" (Alma 5:14.) As you come to the close of this book, do so with this pledge:

> Father, I pledge to you anew my love and my loyalty. I give you my entire self, my body, my free will, my spirit. Help me to live each moment of my present life in your service, consecrating it to you with fervent love.
>
> Without reservation, I also embrace every circumstance of my future—all you have planned for me or will permit me to become, every joy and sorrow, every triumph and failure. Thy will be done.
>
> Likewise, I offer you each moment of my past life. Even my failings, my refusals to serve, my betrayals, I give to you and ask for your forgiveness for all that I should have given you then.
>
> Take, then, my past, my present, and my future, and fuse them into one great whole. Accept me. Strengthen my resolution. Help me to be what you desire.

Please don't close the pages of this book and forget what we have learned together. Use it as a textbook. Refer to it often. Remember that I love you and want you to love yourself.

Go forward with new resolve to stand tall and say to yourself daily:

"There was a queen once . . . and you're looking at her!"

May I Hear from You?

If I can help you in any way, please write to me: Barbara Barrington Jones, Dept. W, 10 Badger Court, Novato, California 94949. If you prefer, you may write in care of the Publishing Department, Deseret Book Company, P. O. Box 30178, Salt Lake City, Utah 84130. Additional copies of this book or of my previous book, *The Inside-Outside Beauty Book,* may be ordered by calling Deseret Book Direct's toll-free number: 1-800-453-4532.

Index